The Complete
Make-up Artist

The Complete Make-up Artist

Working in Film, Fashion, Television and Theatre

Second Edition

Penny Delamar

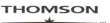

Australia · Canada · Mexico · Singapore · Spain · United Kingdom · United States

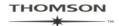

The Complete Make-up Artist – Working in Film, Fashion, Television and Theatre

Copyright © Penny Delamar 2003

The Thomson logo is a registered trademark used herein under licence

For more information, contact Thomson Learning, High Holborn House, 50–51 Bedford Row, London, WC1R 4LR or visit us on the World Wide Web at: http://www.thomsonlearning.co.uk

British Library Cataloguing-in-Publication Data
A catalogue record for this book is available from the British Library

ISBN-13: 978-1-86152-890-6
ISBN-10: 1-86152-890-6

First edition printed by Macmillan, 1995
Second edition published by Thomson, 2003
Reprinted 2005 by Thomson Learning

Typeset by Meridian Colour Repro Ltd, Pangbourne-on-Thames, Berkshire

Printed and bound in Spain by Bookprint S.L., Barcelona

Note on products

The solvents, adhesives and other chemical formulae used in media make-up are constantly changing – new products become available; existing ones are improved; occasionally some are withdrawn from use for reasons of health and safety. You need to know the health and safety regulations, and to be guided by specialist suppliers. This applies particularly in prosthetics. If a product is withdrawn, there is always an improved version or something else which will do the same job. This book refers to products relevant at the time of writing.

The solvent for cleaning brushes is referred to simply as a 'brush cleaner' as the product used has been changed many times. Trichloroethane, used in the past in some medical adhesives and certain brush cleaners, is now known to be one contributor to the depletion of the zone layer; it is likely that in time there will be a total world ban on the use of such products. Nevertheless, manufacturers are researching, improving existing products, and creating new, better and safer products for use in the future.

Provided you use products from a reputable manufacturer and a reputable supply outlet, it is safe to assume that all of the classification, packaging and labelling regulations have been complied with, and that health and safety data sheets will be supplied on request.

Advisory note

Every care has been taken in the writing and editing of this book to ensure that its content is accurate, and that the techniques described and the products referred to are safe when properly used in accordance with professional guidance and/or manufacturers instructions. Training techniques for which special apparatus or chemicals are needed should be undertaken only in the presence of a suitable qualified and experienced teacher. Readers are urged to have due regards to health and safety considerations in applying what is learned. If in doubt, the appropriate professional should be sought. The author and publishers cannot accept legal responsibility for any problems, loss or damage arising from misuse of the methods or products described in the book.

Contents

Foreword

When Penny asked me to contribute to this book, I had for the first time in my career to give serious thought to the relationship between the actor and his or her make-up artist.

The first thing I realised was that, just as it is said that we spend a third of our lives sleeping, so it could be said that an actor may spend up to a third of his or her working day in the make-up chair. For *The Elephant Man*, for example, John Hurt spent something like five hours a day having grotesque, elephantine features superimposed on his own face. Once, while filming in Rome, I spent two hours every morning sitting in the make-up chair with a *Teach Yourself Italian* book, listening to the Italian conversation around me. When, after three months, the filming ended, my Italian was almost fluent.

The make-up artist is someone with whom we actors spend a lot of time. So, to the huge meal of knowledge and experience Penny is offering you in this book, I'd like to add a pinch of psychology.

You, the make-up artist, are often the first person the actor sees at the early start of a long working day. If an actor is depressed, ill, nervous or going through a divorce, you will be the first to know. The face looking up at you from the make-up chair will tell you everything. If the actor *says* nothing, you will need to be a sensitive mind-reader; if she or he needs to *talk*, you'll need to be a discreet listener and confidante – no matter how boring you may find it!

The actor's face is his or her mask, and that – literally – is what is in your hands. Actors need you to understand their mental picture of the characters they are playing; your skill will help to make that image a reality. Then they can project their characters with complete conviction, confident that they *look* as they feel.

When all is said and done, when all the preparation is complete, finally it is the actor who stands in front of the camera to deliver the goods, seeking to please producers and audience alike. That is a weighty responsibility: it can put a lot of strain on someone. If an actor is rude, there's no excuse; but should he or she be irritable or difficult, never take it personally. Remember that in an industry where time equals money, people feel the pressure.

I'm not saying that your career as a make-up artist will be filled solely with actors sharing their life's woes or throwing tantrums. On the contrary, in the world of film and TV, which is unique, I assure you there'll be a lot of laughs. In fact, it's the laughs that keep the wind in everyone's sails and get through long weeks of long days of shooting.

So, when you pack your kit and put in your sable brushes, your sponges, foundations and powder puffs, don't forget to pack your sense of humour – it's a crucial part of your equipment.

Cherie Lunghi

Introduction

The role of the make-up artist

In her Foreword to this book the actress, Cherie Lunghi, describes beautifully the role of the make-up artist from an actor's point of view. It is certainly true that all actors gravitate towards the make-up room, where tea and sympathy are dispensed in equal proportions. Maintaining a happy atmosphere is as much a part of the job as the technical skills of make-up.

In order to get a broader picture of the role of the make-up artist I have consulted a variety of professionals, with different levels of experience. The result is a series of artists' profiles that appear throughout this book, allowing us valuable insights into their individual careers. You will notice that these profiles all have one thing in common. From Oscar winners to trainees, they are all passionate about the quality of their work.

In these uncertain times, with computers replacing people in many areas of work, we can be confident that machines will never replace the make-up artists. Once learned, make-up is a skill that cannot be taken from you – a worthwhile possession in the changing fortunes of modern times.

Penny Delamar

Penny Delamar

Website: www.themake-upcentre.co.uk
Email: info@themake-upcentre.co.uk

Acknowledgements

I would like to thank the following people and organisations for their assistance in producing this book:

Luisa Abel
James Anda
Joyce Allsworth
Live Karine Appelland
Desmond Barritt
Christine Blundell
Cecilia Blomstedt
Rebecca Burge
Lois Burwell
Tricia Cameron
Katherine Colson
Charlotte Cowen
Marie de la Motte
Sonia Farhadi
Kevin Fortune
Jane Fox
Alex Frost
Jo Frost
Charmaine Fuller
Eleonara Giampieri
Louise Goldman
Hiroe Goto
Charlotte Greenwood
Siobhan Harper Ryan
Miles Hawkins
Poppy Hill
Francesca Hingston
Susanna Humbel
May Walid Abdel Jabbar
Sarah Jagger
Stephanie Kelly
Julie Kendrick
Brian Kinney
Julia Laderman
Ken Lintott
Cherie Lunghi
Debbie Mackay

Louise McCarthy
Jessica McLeod
Liz Michie
Agata Do Miguelle
Linda Morton
Caroline O'Connor
Joanne O'Keefe
Michelle O'Neil
Pam Orange
Conor O'Sullivan
Shauna O'Toole
Jane Powell
Christine Powers
Trefor Proud
Meineer Rees
Gemma Richards
Jacqueline Russon
Dolly Ryan
Jolanta Sewell
Stuart Sewell
Kulwadee Songsiri
Leda Shawyer
Tom Smith
Sally Studley
Simona Stutz
Camilla Tew
Akiko Toida
Anna Tyndale Biscoe
Louisa Ward
Jason Weihov
Wig Specialities
Julia Wilson
Marion Wilson
Helen Wix

Photographers Nigel Tribbeck, Simon Warren, Holly Warburton

Lord Attenborough for photographs taken by Frank Conner from *Ghandi*, an Indo-British Films Production.

Mike Leigh for photographs from *Topsy Turvy* of Timothy Spall, Martin Savage, Katrin Cartlidge, Allan Corduner, Cathy Sara, Shirley Henderson and Dorothy Atkinson.

Katherine Dore, Les Brotherston and Mathew Bourne for photographs from *The Car Man* and *Swan Lake*.

Granada Television for photographs from *Night and Day*.

Last, but by no means least, many thanks to all the make-up artists and models who were involved in the various technique photographs taken for this book, and for contributing their case profiles as examples to students of make-up.

Thanks are also due to my family, David, Leda, Leonora and Gideon, for their contribution and support. Special thanks go to Salma Bhurtun for her patience and expertise in preparing my new manuscript.

Media make-up as a career

Introduction

The freelance make-up artist

Years ago the film and television studios used to employ permanent staff, but those days are long gone. Some theatres, such as the English National Opera and the Royal National Theatre, still have make-up artists on staff as well as employing freelancers to assist with busy productions. So do a few television companies, usually to make up the news announcers and programme presenters. Apart from these exceptions, all the available work in film, television, music videos and fashion is freelance. A freelancer is a one-person business and will usually employ an accountant to sort out their tax liability at the end of the year. Although it sounds insecure, the freelance make-up artist often winds up working for the same few companies or photographers for several years. A film or television designer will often use the same make-up artist to assist them whenever possible, so being freelance is not as lonely as it sounds. At the beginning it is difficult because it takes time to become known and established in the industry. It is important to have a CV and portfolio (and later on even a show reel) to demonstrate to potential employers that you are confident in your skills.

Like all self-employed people, you will need a mobile phone and the flexibility to be available for meetings and work at all times. There are many 'answer service' agencies and 'diary' companies for TV and film crews. They provide information on jobs and keep a record of work availability for make-up artists and other crew personnel on their books in return for a monthly payment. Fashion make-up artists always use agents, and top film make-up designers also have agents who look after their contracts and fees. However, none of these agencies will take on anyone until they have a proven track record. When starting off it is from other make-up artists that you will get a foothold in the TV, film and theatre industries.

Areas of specialisation for long-term progression

To begin with, a young make-up artist is better off accepting every experience that comes their way, whether in fashion, theatre, TV or film. Eventually, either through choice or circumstance, they will settle into one of these areas in order to make a living. For example, if early morning calls at 5am are impossible for you, then perhaps working in theatre would be easier, since the make-up artists do matinee and evening performances. If wig styling is not your favourite occupation then you will have to forget theatre. If someone really wants to break into fashion then they have to do test shots and find an agent. Eventually everyone settles into the niche they prefer. There are some specialisations that are niche areas, and production companies and make-up artists hire their services when needed:

- manufacturing wigs
- manufacturing facial hair
- manufacturing prosthetics
- manufacturing bald caps
- body painting
- bridal make-up
- camouflage in private clinics
- make-up in beauty salons
- teaching and writing
- children's face-painting
- consultations and individual make-up lessons.

These specialist people may not advertise their services widely – but they used to do hair/make-up in TV and films and then decided to set up on their own at home. Other make-up artists commission their work and soon the specialist is working as much as they want – at home or in a workshop.

If someone wants to provide a specialist shop with their bald caps or prosthetic pieces, they can approach any of the professional make-up supplier shops. For a percentage, these shops will sell their products. There are even make-up artists who make and distribute their own artificial blood.

Creating cosmetic product lines is also an option later on – but the make-up artist needs to be well known and probably from fashion in order to compete with the numerous well-known brands.

Bridal make-up is a specialisation that any make-up artist can combine with a home life and family quite easily. All it takes is an advertisement placed in bridal magazines or a good website to tell everyone you are available.

For the make-up artist who is tired of years of early calls and foreign locations, there is teaching. Rather than giving up make-up, it is satisfying to pass your skills on to the next generation. Then there is writing, which also can be done at home in your own time, albeit to strict deadlines.

In the 1960s a film make-up artist called Dave Aylott started making eyelashes and created the company Eyelure. You can still buy the company's eyelashes in any chemist shop. He made a fortune.

Portfolios

Make-up artists usually use a portfolio the size of a tear sheet – A4. Your portfolio should reflect the work you have done and the type of work you wish to do. For work in film, TV and theatre you should display everything that a well-rounded make-up artist can do, i.e. beauty and straight make-up, ageing, character, facial hair, wigs, bald cap, casualty, prosthetics, etc., plus your CV.

For work in fashion and editorial, your portfolio should have beauty and fashion pictures, plus your CV. It is not a good idea to include photographs showing make-up artists being cuddled by actors; this reflects the make-up artists' egos – not their work. Choose pictures for their quality. It is better to have a few good ones than too many of inferior quality. As your work increases you will be constantly updating your portfolio and discarding out-of-date pictures. You can improve your portfolio on a computer, adjusting the colour, removing scratches, tidying up stray hairs that are out of place, or removing a cluttered background.

Never use a photo in your portfolio of someone else's work, or a credit on your CV that is false. Not only is this morally and professionally wrong, but you will always get caught out. Remember that 'before' and 'after' pictures are good to have in your portfolio because they show off your work, particularly subtle make-ups.

The role of the trainee make-up artist

It is a well-known fact that you do not learn to drive until you have passed your driving test. The same could be said of make-up artistry. When you have successfully graduated from college you need to obtain work experience on professional productions. The way to do this is to contact make-up artists and ask them to take you on as a trainee for a day, a week or a month. If the tutors on your course are working make-up artists, they may be able to place you with a colleague. You need as much work experience as you can get in the first year after graduation. Every job, however small, will always lead to others and you never know who you will meet or what contacts you will make. Trainees are paid a minimal amount, usually only enough to survive, but this should be looked upon as a continuation of the training process, since that is what it is. It should also be done with enthusiasm. The make-up artist in charge will expect you to be a runner or gofer (go for this, go for that), to assist the rest of the team, get the coffee, clean the make-up places, check the stockroom and perhaps do make-ups when there are crowd artists on busy days. Above all – always be on time, ready to start work, with a smile.

Never think that being a runner is inferior work. It is not, so do everything with a good grace. When running errands you will meet members of other departments and begin to understand their roles. You will gain contacts with other make-up artists on crowd calls and learn about make-up products when sorting out the stockroom. When you clean other make-up artists' work stations, you will learn a great deal about how the make-up was applied – particularly beards, moustaches, wigs and prosthetics. Every make-up artist started this way; we have all been there.

On your training course you were the customer, with experienced make-up artists teaching you and considering your needs. Now you will be expected to anticipate the make-up designers' needs. So watch, listen and learn. In quiet moments you can be taught about lighting, lenses and continuity. But do not ask questions when people are busy, do not stand talking to other crew members when a make-up artist needs your assistance and, above all, do everything you are asked straightaway and with good will. Attitude is everything.

The make-up room

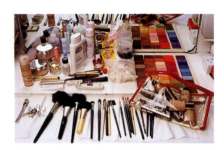

Tools of the trade

The working area

Make-up rooms in film studios, television studios and theatres are custom-built to provide the necessary working surfaces, lighting and storage facilities: it is easy to move in and prepare the working environment. *On location* and on small-budget productions, however, this is often not the case: the surroundings may be uncomfortable, cramped and ill-equipped. In such situations it is the make-up artist's job to establish the working area.

- **The room** The room allocated should be well ventilated to meet health and safety regulations.
- **The facilities** There should be a mirror, a table and lights for each make-up artist. Electricity points must be adequate and checked prior to use. Close at hand there should be a washbasin with hot and cold running water.
- **The environment** The temperature and humidity must be comfortable for working and stable for the storage of make-up materials.

If such ideal conditions are not available, it is essential to notify the location manager or production office promptly and to state clearly what is required.

Health and hygiene

Once the working area has been transformed into a make-up room, it is up to the make-up artist to maintain a *safe*, *healthy* and *hygienic* working environment to safeguard both colleagues and models from accident and infection. Provided that you take sensible precautions, the make-up room can be kept safe and clean.

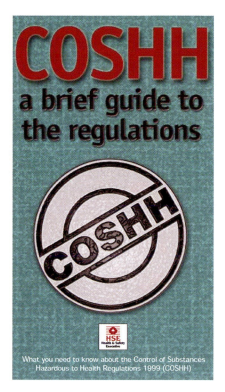

COSHH Employers Guide

Cross-contamination via make-up

Infections, such as scabies, cold sores, styes and other viral and bacterial diseases, can be spread via sponges, powder puffs, foundations, creams, lipstick and so on. Such diseases can also be passed on via equipment that has not been sterilised or cleaned properly. For this reason, and also because the acids in your skin could contaminate the make-up, you should not touch make-up products with your hands. Instead, use spatulas and brushes.

Control of Substances Hazardous to Health (COSHH) 1988

The COSHH 1988 regulations provide guidance and lay down rules about the safe storage and use of potentially dangerous substances. You should be familiar with these regulations. A copy of the COSSH regulations can be obtained from the office of your local Health and Safety Executive (HSE). In particular you should know about the correct storage and use of cleaning agents and ensure that the storage area is clearly identified.

Working hygienically

General preparations

- **Make-up products** should always be labelled clearly, with full instructions for use. This is to avoid accidents, such as mistaking surgical spirit or acetone for skin tonic.
- **Hazardous materials** should be kept securely, in lockable cabinets or metal trunks.
- **Wraps and towels** must always be clean and freshly laundered.
- **Individual make-up boxes** should be cleaned out regularly.
- **Electrical sockets and plugs** must be safe. If any are faulty, get them repaired immediately.
- **Tools** must be sterilised. Clean electrical equipment such as shavers, beard trimmers, tongs, electric hair curlers and the like using surgical spirit. (Always follow manufacturers' instructions.)
- **Mirrors** should be kept polished.

Before starting the make-up

- Check that you have clean powder puffs, sponges and brushes to hand.

While working

- When applying lipstick, use a *spatula* to transfer the lipstick onto a *palette*. (A ceramic tile serves as an inexpensive palette.) Then use a clean *lipbrush* to apply the lip colour from the palette.

When you have finished

- As soon as the make-up has been completed, clean any brushes in *brush-cleaning solvent*.
- *Sponges* and *powder puffs* should be washed and sterilised, or thrown away if they are particularly dirty (as they will be if they have been used for special effects work or heavy character make-up).
- Dispose of *solvent removers* safely, in covered bins.
- At the end of the working day, *work surfaces* should be scrubbed down and the floor swept.

Professionalism

The make-up artist who always behaves professionally will be more successful than the one who does not. The best time to develop this professionalism is while you are training. The make-up room should be a haven of calm. Models and actors need a restful atmosphere, away from the hustle and bustle of the set. The make-up artist may be the last person they speak to before going in front of the camera. It is vital that the make-up artist is unflustered in her work. Often the director's assistant will be urgently asking 'How much longer will you be?' or telling you to 'Hurry up', but you must not be distracted by such pressures.

Efficient working

It will be easier to remain calm and purposeful if you are well organised and your working area is clean and tidy. If everything is laid out ready when the model arrives, not only is this more pleasant but it also saves time.

Storing materials

- **Kit boxes** Keep separate kit boxes for straight make-up, casualty effects and hairdressing. Inexpensive boxes intended for tools or fishing tackle are quite adequate.
- **Storage** Store materials in such a way that they will not be damaged, crushed, spilt or broken. Store separately any potentially messy materials such as artificial blood, glycerine and dirt.
- **Containers** Plastic bottles are often preferable to glass ones, but make sure that the material concerned can be safely stored in a plastic bottle. This is particularly important for substances such as surgical spirit, isopropyl alcohol and cleaning solvents.

Routine checks

- **Stock** Check your make-up stock regularly so that you do not run out of materials. Refill bottles as necessary. Report any needs to the production office.
- **Cleaning** Check that you have sufficient cleaning and sterilising fluids, appropriate to the materials you are using. (This is especially important when working on location.)
- **Labels** Ensure that the labels on all bottles and jars are clear and accurate.

Ordering materials

- **Avoiding waste** When purchasing materials for a production, take care that the products are suitable and economical. Don't use expensive brands for crowd scenes in which the actors will not be seen in close-up.
- **Special needs** Do any of the actors or models have special skin-care needs?
- **Getting quotes** When ordering facial hair and prosthetics, hiring or buying wigs, get quotes from several suppliers. The cheapest may not be the best quality, but at least consider the options.
- **Keeping records** Keep clear and accurate records of transactions. Notify production promptly of expenses incurred.

Working abroad

- **Air freight** If you need to have materials sent by air freight, arrange this in advance. Make sure that products are packed carefully to avoid breakages.

Clothing

- **Planning ahead** Be sure that you have sensible and appropriate clothing for the weather conditions that you may encounter where you are working.

Continuity

- **Keeping reference materials** To ensure continuity, make notes, charts and sketches to record your work and take Polaroid photographs as necessary. These can be kept in a file or pinned to the wall so that you can refer to them as you work.

Personal appearance

Be discreet with your choice of clothing and jewellery – the artiste, not the make-up artist, is the 'star'! Maintain high standards of personal hygiene:

- Keep long hair tied back off the face.
- Do not use too much make-up on your own face: the artistes might think that you would also apply too much make-up to them!
- Wear flat-soled shoes – high heels can cause accidents in the studio.
- Do not smoke in the make-up room.
- Keep your fingernails scrupulously clean and reasonably short. Long fingernails are dangerous and make application of make-up difficult.

Working on set

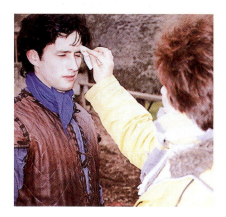

A make-up artist at work

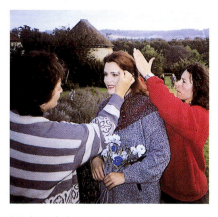

Maintaining make-up

When the make-up is completed and the actor is on the set, your responsibility has not ended. It is now necessary to maintain the make-up you have applied, so that it remains intact throughout the shoot. Whether working inside the studio under hot lights or outside on location in various weather conditions, it is important to stand by, ready to repair any damage to the make-up.

The make-up artist should have all the necessary tools and materials in a *small bag* or *set box*. Clear *plastic bags with zip fastenings* are useful: these not only protect your materials but make it easy to recognise them at a glance. As the set is usually dirty, perhaps with smoke machines and other effects being used, avoid leaving your kit box open or uncovered.

Check the make-up between shots, with a complete check after each meal break. Touching up includes adding more lipstick, blotting perspiration, and repowdering. Even if you are simply blotting perspiration with a cleaning tissue or adding lipstick, it is advisable to encourage the actor to sit comfortably in a chair. When the actor needs a complete change of costume, hair and make-up, you must make arrangements with the assistant director to allow time for this.

Whether repairing the make-up or applying a new one for reasons of continuity, it is always essential to move quickly yet remain calm. The work should be done without holding up the production.

Team work

To an outsider it always looks as if everyone on the set is hanging around doing nothing. This is because everyone else has to wait whilst someone finishes his or her work. Lights need adjusting, props must be moved and tracks must be laid down for the cameras to move on. All these activities take time, so whenever you have work to do, you need to do it immediately, as others may be waiting for you.

The make-up artist should never leave the set without first informing another member of the make-up team or an assistant director. Unexpected things happen all the time: if the set is left unattended, the make-up artist is sure to be needed at that moment!

There are many potential hazards on the set, such as trailing cables and wires: to avoid accidents, always wear sensible flat shoes with rubber soles. Don't wear anything that makes a noise such as jangling bracelets or squeaky footwear: any such sound can hold up the work.

The entire crew work closely together and by being sympathetic towards one another they create a good team. Everyone relies on the others to work well, efficiently and fast. When working under pressure in this way it is vital to establish good working relationships with everyone involved. Since intense pressure is normal on a shoot, and indeed necessary to generate the required energy, the professional make-up artist must learn to cope with stress. Consideration towards the actors, such as providing them with coffee at the right moment, can help greatly in alleviating their tension.

A useful item to carry when working on the set is a good-quality *chamois leather*. This can be soaked in cold water, squeezed until damp and then sprinkled with cologne. When twirled in the air, the leather becomes ice-cold. If an actor is excessively hot you can relieve the symptoms by placing the chamois leather at the back of his neck to cool him down, which in turn helps to maintain the make-up. Small *battery fans* are also good for keeping actors cool.

Background study

Many other subjects provide a good basis for a career in make-up. *Drawing, painting, sculpting, hairdressing* and *history of art* are clearly relevant; *chemistry* is useful as preparation for working in prosthetics. For artists who wish to be able to pursue their careers across Europe and the rest of the world, *foreign languages* are always invaluable. An understanding of facial anatomy is also important. In order to understand how to improve or change the appearance of a face, it is vital that you understand the *bone structure* beneath the flesh.

The skull

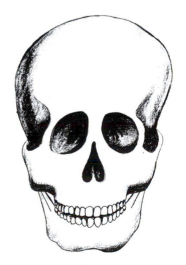

A study of the human skull is the first lesson in the approach to make-up.

 Activity – Drawing the skull

1 Using a soft lead pencil, draw the skull on white paper, noting the darkest and lightest areas.
2 Draw the skull again, this time marking in the technical names of the bones.

Lighting and shading

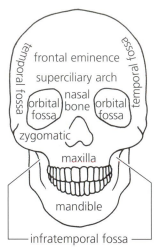

temporal fossa

frontal eminence

superciliary arch

nasal bone

orbital fossa

orbital fossa

temporal fossa

zygomatic

maxilla

mandible

infratemporal fossa

The bones of the face

Tip

When drawing shaded areas, use your finger to smudge the edges and so produce a soft effect.

Now that you have a basic understanding of the structure of the human skull, it is time to examine a real face – looking at and feeling the bones beneath the flesh.

Activity – Studying a face

You will need: a fellow student to work with and two brushes – one for black, the other for white; two make-up colours, either cream or water-based.

1 Using your colleague as a model, feel the prominences and depressions on the entire face.
2 Paint in the hollows of the face with black and the prominent areas with white.

At the end, your model's face will resemble the skull you have been studying.

Faces and head shapes

Both make-up and hair should be designed to suit the model's head and face shape. There are seven basic face shapes.

The oval face

This is generally considered to be the perfect shape – it is easy to work on and photographs well.

The round face

This shape needs slimming. Shading with make-up at the sides of the face will help. The hairstyle should not be full at the sides as that would emphasise the round shape. Instead, dress the hair high at the front or straight down at the sides to minimise the jawline.

The long face

This shape can be shaded at the chin, which shortens the apparent length. Blusher can be placed on the apples of cheeks to give the illusion of a rounder shape. Hair can be dressed full at the sides to add width.

The square face

This should be shaded at the jawline to soften the appearance. Blusher can be placed high on the cheekbones, defining their shape, or shaded underneath for a slimming effect.

The heart-shaped face

With this shape, blusher should be placed on the round apples of the cheeks. No shading should be used except at the sides of the

Different face shapes

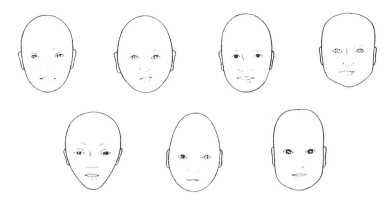

forehead close to the hairline. The shape can be balanced by a hairstyle that is full at the jawline.

The pear-shaped face

This is the opposite to the heart-shaped face, with the head being narrower at the top and the bottom half of the face being more rounded in shape. Definition can be added by shading to slim the sides of the face, working from below the cheekbones. The hairstyle should be designed to add width and height at the top of the head.

The rectangular face

In this case shading and contouring can be used at the sides of the face, especially at the jawline. The hair should not be high at the top, but used to soften the shape, with forward hair movements and fullness at the sides.

Facial structure

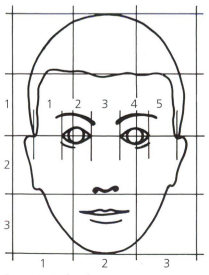

Skull make-up

The best way to understand the structure of the face is to draw it on paper. Before you start, bear in mind the following:

1   Note the *type of head* and the *shape of face* – round, long, square, oval, etc.
2   Consider the person's *character* – the expression, the set of the features and the relation of each feature to the others. These aspects determine the model's liveliness, humour, pensiveness and so on in the sketch.
3   Look out for anything *unusual* about the face you are drawing – a distinctive nose perhaps, or a prominent chin, jaw or lower lip. Draw what you see.

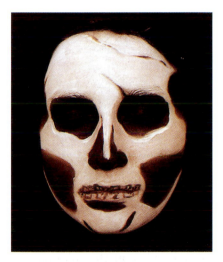

Drawing the face

 Activity – Drawing the face (1)

Take pencil and paper and begin by drawing the face of a fellow student, or looking in a mirror and drawing yourself.

The main errors made by the beginner usually are to set the eyes too high – they should be about halfway down the length of the face – and getting the eyes slightly out of line with each other. Note that the face can be divided horizontally:

- from the hairline to the centre of the eyes
- from the eyes to the tip of the nose
- from the tip of the nose to the chin

The eyes consist of two semicircles, the upper one being slightly wider in diameter and more curved than the lower. The eyes can be used to measure five areas from side to side:

- the eyes themselves
- the space between the eyes
- the two spaces between the outer corners of the eyes and the hairline at the edge of the face

Between the eye and the eyebrow there is roughly an eye's depth of space. Of course, shapes and measurements vary considerably between individuals. The shape of the nose, for instance, varies enormously. It can be paralled sided or wedge shaped, thinnest at the bridge and widest at the nostrils.

When you draw the mouth, make certain that you place it so that the length of the chin and the length of the space between the end of the nose and the top lip are both correct. The bottom lip is usually fuller than the top one; the top lip is normally wider than the bottom one.

The ears are usually the same length as the nose. When viewed from the front, the top of the ear is normally in line with the bridge of the nose and the ear lobe in line with the tip of the nose.

 Activity – Drawing the face (2)

1 Take it in turns to draw one another's faces from the front. Try always to achieve a good likeness.
2 Measure the relative distances and the proportions by holding your pencil between your eye and the face you are sketching. Transfer these measurements to your paper.
3 Sketch your model's face from the side, observing the profile and shape of the brow ridge, the cheekbone, the nose, the mouth and the chin.

Remember, you are not attempting a work of art, but an exercise in accurate observation and in drawing what you see.

Activity – Drawing a square on the face

This is an exercise to help students co-ordinate brains, eyes and hands. It is not as easy as it would seem at first. Since the face is contoured, it is necessary to use curves instead of a straight lines on the cheek areas. The model should face the mirror whilst you work it out.

Paint the outline of the square using a white watercolour, as it is easy to clean off and start again, rather than black pencil which is harder to remove. When the outline is perfect you can then paint the space in your preferred colour.

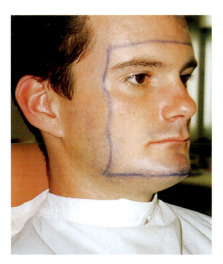

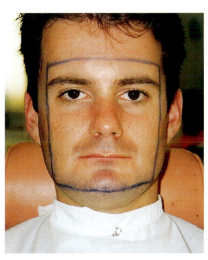

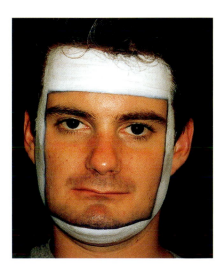

**Drawing a square on the face
Side view**

Front view

Final effect

Colour

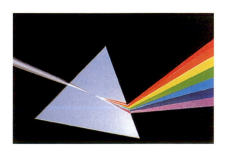

The colour spectrum

A real understanding of colour is absolutely basic for the make-up artist.

Principles of colour

The colours we see depend on the colour of the *light source*, the colours of any *filters* used and the colour of the *objects* that then *reflect* the light.

In the retina at the back of the eye, there are two kinds of receptor cells: these respond to light focused on them by the lens of the eye. One sort is responsible for colourless vision in dim light and the other for colour perception in bright light.

White light is a mixture of light of many different wavelengths. If you shine a beam of white light through a glass prism, the rays are bent according to their wavelengths and spread out to form a multicoloured *spectrum*. The spectrum can be seen if a screen is placed in its path. The order of the colours is always the same, the order that you see in a rainbow: violet, indigo, blue, green, yellow, orange and red.

When white light strikes a white surface, most of the light is *reflected*, which is why the surface looks white. When light strikes a black surface, most of it is *absorbed*. When light strikes a grey or coloured surface, some is reflected and some is absorbed. When white light strikes a red surface, for example, the surface appears red because it is reflecting red light, but absorbing light of other colours. When light strikes a transparent surface, most of it simply passes through.

From a technical point of view, make-up and paint pigments have no colour of their own: they seem coloured to us because they absorb light of some wavelengths and reflect light of others. The light reflected produces the particular colour we see.

Classifying colour

Colours are classified in three ways: according to their *hue*, their *brightness* and their *intensity*.

Hue

The hue of a colour represents the difference between pure colours – the name by which we know it: red, blue, yellow, and so forth.

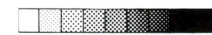

The scale of greys

Brightness

Brightness represents the range from light to dark. From any light colour to any dark colour there is a brightness scale. The scale of greys is simple because there are no hues.

The darkness or lightness of a colour – its position on the range – is called its *value*. A *light* colour has *high* value while a *dark* colour has a *low* value.

Intensity

Intensity is the range from any pure hue to a point of the grey scale. A grey-blue, for example, has a blue hue, yet is different from the pure blue of the colour wheel. Although it is of the same hue (blue), it is lower in intensity. It is nearer to the centre of the wheel, and more grey. The colours on the outside of the wheel are brilliant. Those nearer the centre of the wheel are less brilliant and known as *tones*. Intensity scales are of three kinds:

- **tints**, ranging from any pure hue to white
- **shades**, ranging from any pure hue to black
- **tones**, ranging from any pure hue to a grey

Each hue can be produced by mixing some combination of the three primary colours: red, yellow and blue. Variations can be made by adding black, white or both. Similarly, you can change make-up foundation colours by mixing them. If a colour is not warm enough, add some red. If it is too dark, add some white. If it looks too bright, add some grey (which you make by mixing black and white).

 Activity – Matching colours (1)

1 By mixing watercolour paints, experiment in the matching of colours. Aim to mix a particular tint, shade or tone. At first you will find it difficult, but with practice you will improve rapidly.

2 Mix different flesh tones. Once you have produced several, write down the proportions of colours used, then mix the same colours again.

Never rely on the *description* of a make-up colour. 'Chinese yellow' is not suitable for all Chinese people, for example. 'Indian' is not automatically going to be the right base for a native of India. Train your eye to judge colours accurately. Good make-up relies on your knowledge and your ability to assess colour.

 Activity – Matching colours (2)

Select three foundation colours and try to match them, using red, yellow, blue, black and white panstiks.

The colour circle

The colour circle or colour wheel used by artists and decorators for distinguishing colours can also be applied to makeup colours, which are paints for the face.

- **Primary paint colours** Red, blue and yellow, when mixed in equal proportions, produce *grey*.
- **Secondary paint colours** Orange, green and violet are each made by mixing two adjacent primary colours.
- **In-between colours** Made by mixing more of one colour than another, for example, bluish green or greenish blue.
- **Tints** Made by adding white – this can produce colours such as opal.
- **Shades** Made by adding black – this can produce colours such as emerald.

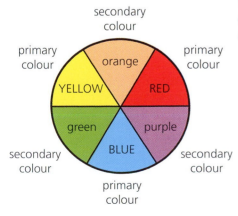

The colour circle

Colour co-ordination

It is important that the make-up artist is careful to select and match products that co-ordinate – that is, colours that relate to one another in the completed make-up.

- **Foundation** The foundation should match the skin colour.
- **Eyebrows** The eyebrow pencil or powder should match the hair colour, or at least harmonise with it. For example, a person with ash blonde hair would need her eyebrows defined with taupe, which is a pale grey brown. If instead you used other shades of brown, such as browns with red in them, this would look wrong. A brown with ginger tones would look correct on a red-headed person.
- **Cheeks** In women's make-up, blusher or rouge should be harmonious with the skin tone. It should not be treated as an accessory to match the dress.
- **Lips** Lip colour should be considered in relation to the costume, as well as in relation to the skin tone and the hair.
- **Eyes** Eye colours should improve or define the eyes as well as harmonising with the total look and style.

Making the most of colour

There are thousands of colours in the world around us. However many colours you may have in your make-up box, you will almost certainly need to mix some of them in order to create the colours you need.

Mixing colours

The cleanest, clearest colours come straight from the pot, box or tube. Mixed with other colours they become muddy. As a general rule, *it is best to mix no more than two colours together*, though the result can be modified with a spot of another colour.

Primary and secondary colours

The *primary colours* in make-up are blue, red and yellow.

- blue mixed with yellow gives a series of greens, from bluish green (more blue than yellow) to a pale, yellowish green (more yellow than blue)
- red mixed with yellow gives a full range of oranges
- red mixed with blue gives a range of purples

Green, orange and purple are *secondary colours*. The hues of the primary colours from which they are mixed will have a large effect on the result.

Making the most of colour

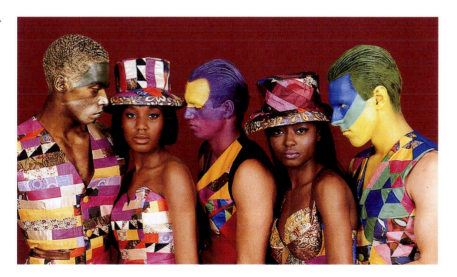

Adding white

Pastel shades such as delicate pinks, blues, greens, apricots, creams and lilacs – can be made by adding white to red, blue, green, orange, yellow or purple. If you add too much white, the colour will look chalky.

Adding black

The addition of black will create a *shade* of any given colour. It will dull any pigment you mix it with, however, and should therefore be used with caution. Mixed with yellow ochre, it makes a pleasant olive green.

Adding grey

Black and white together give tones of grey. By themselves, these are cold; add a touch of yellow, brown or red to warm the colour.

Complementary and harmonising colours

Each colour has a *complementary colour*, diametrically opposite it on the colour wheel. When any two complementary colours are placed next to each other, they produce a strong contrast and each of the colours looks more vivid.

Colours that share a pigment, such as blue and green, are called *harmonising colours*: when placed next to each other they appear to blend.

If you stare long and hard at a particular colour (say, red) and then look hard at a white surface, you may see an after-image of the complementary colour (in the case of red, green). This is because the eye has ceased to register the original colour and is now registering the remaining colours in the mixture that makes up white light. This explains why it is so hard to match colours. After comparing many different samples for a long time, your brain ceases to register the correct colour. Complementary colours can be used in make-up in the following ways:

- **Toning down** A colour can be toned down by adding a little of the complementary colour. Thus, a too-bright red can be toned down by adding a touch of green (and vice versa).
- **Making greyer** Any colour can be made greyer by adding a small quantity of its complementary colour.

Neutral or earth colours

These are blacks, greys and browns. You will make an earth colour if you mix together:

- the three primary colours
- any two secondary colours
- all the primary and secondary colours

Guidelines in using colour

Don't be tempted to use too many bright colours in one make-up as the result could be discordant. Using one or two pure colours can help to create a focal point on the face, but more than that will confuse. The eye will pass from one bright colour to the other and, because there is no contrast between brighter and more muted colours, the colours will fight for attention.

Not all cool colours are dull and not all warm colours are bright. There are dull reds and yellows, and bright blues and greens. Whether cool or warm, dull or intense, the mood can be determined by colour.

Don't worry about matching colour exactly. It is more important to get the *tonal differences* right – the degree of darkness or lightness of colours in relation to each other. Consider a black-and-white photograph. Which are the dark, medium and light areas?

Skin care

Specialist skin care belongs to the world of beauty therapy. As make-up artists apply make-up, beauticians make their living from caring for their clients' skin. There are an enormous number of skin treatment creams, available from many companies, devoted to cleansing, toning, buffing, soothing, peeling or massaging. Very often the beauty therapist has a connection with a particular beauty product company and does her treatments with and sells a particular line of products.

Beauty therapists also provide services in dyeing eyelashes and removing unwanted hair on the face or body by plucking, waxing, sugaring, bleaching or electrolysis. They are trained in giving aromatherapy and other massage treatments, plus thread vein treatments, manicures and pedicures. This is a highly skilled and specialist area of work – not the make-up artists' field at all – though many beauticians do go on to train as make-up artists.

Most people visit a beautician for skin treatments, with actors and models more regular clients than the average person. They are usually keenly aware of their appearance because 'their faces are their fortunes' and have to be maintained at all costs. Not only do they regularly visit their favourite hairdressers for colouring, cutting and styling, but they also have their favourite beauticians, dentists, opticians and fitness trainers. The make-up artist is responsible for putting make-up on faces to look good for the cameras and making sure that the skin is restored to its original state when the make-up is removed. Cleansers, toners and moisturisers should always be available in the make-up room, even though most professional performers have their personal skin-care preparations.

Most damage to the skin is not caused by make-up or skin-care products, but by rough treatment when removing make-up too quickly. It is therefore important for make-up artists to have the correct removing oil or cream when they have used spirit gum or other bonding agents for prosthetics, facial hair and wigs. Most of the companies producing products to apply to the skin also supply the correct products to remove them.

Most actresses have their own cleansing routine and it is not the make-up artist's job to look after their skin. However, on a long film or television series the actors' skin problems do concern the make-up artists, because the skin is the canvas on which they paint. It is therefore in everyone's interests to make sure that the skin is clean before and after make-up is applied.

Skin structure

The skin consists of three layers:

1 **the epidermis** – the outer layer, which we can see.
2 **the dermis** – the middle skin layer.
3 **the subcutaneous** – the deepest skin layer.

The *subcutaneous* layer protects the body and varies in thickness between one part of the body and another. It insulates against heat and cold and also determines the contours of the face and body.

The *dermis*, which is the middle layer, connects the epidermis and subcutaneous layers with fibrous tissues of collagen and elastin, which is called connective tissue. This is the live part where new cells are formed to replace the old ones which rise to the outer surface and shed themselves as dead skin cells. The dermis contains the nerve endings and sweat glands, which regulate how we feel pain, and the sebaceous glands, which hold the hair roots. The dermis also houses the cells that manufacture melanin, which lets the skin go brown when exposed to the sun.

The *epidermis*, the skin layer we see on the outside, forms the body's first defence against infection. As the cells rise to the epidermis layer, they die and form a hard surface on the outer skin.

The skin is waterproof. If water is placed on the skin it evaporates. When soap and water are used to clean it, they only wash away the natural fats and oils on the surface. The skin is soft and elastic when young, and after puberty may become greasier, due to increased hormonal activity which sometimes leads to an inbalance of glandular secretions. If the sebaceous glands are producing too much sebum, it can cause the condition known as acne. After puberty the skin may have dry or greasy patches and it is common to have an oily area on the centre of the face with blocked pores. This often results in spots around the nose, chin and forehead.

People with dry skin tend to develop wrinkles in later life due to a lack of moisture. The sun has damaging effects on all skin types, but the dry-skinned person will suffer most. The different types of skin surface are called *normal*, *oily*, *dry* and *combination*. Our skin types are determined by our genes and we inherit our skin type from one or other of our parents.

Cleansing

All skin types have the same need for thorough cleansing, which should penetrate the pores to stop dirt reaching below the epidermis. The cleansing should be done with oil as water does not reach into the pores. Soap, which is alkaline, mixed with water, only cleans the surface of the skin. After washing with normal soap and water the skin feels tight. This tightness does not indicate cleanliness, but is actually a feeling of dryness and the need for oil.

The correct way to clean the skin is to use a water in oil cream, without fragrance, all over the face and then to remove it with damp cottonwool. This is the best method of cleaning the skin, including oily skin types. The cream will trap the skin's own moisture inside, which is also the function of a moisturiser.

Toning

Toners usually consist mostly of water with an added fragrance and often have alcohol in them, which is not beneficial to the skin. Pure rosewater mixed with distilled water and a small amount of glycerine is the best toner for the skin and the least expensive. The toner is used to remove traces of cleansing cream and to close the pores. In actual fact the toner is not capable of penetrating the pores and will merely dry the skin's surface. Toner should be applied and removed with damp cottonwool, which can be thrown away.

Moisturising

Moisturisers are used to put moisture back into the skin after cleansing. A small amount should be placed on clean fingertips with a spatula and gently patted all over the face, without dragging the skin downwards. All movements of the cleansing, toning and moisturising procedures should be upwards.

Effects of lighting

Effects of lighting on make-up

Whether you are working in photography, theatre, television or film, the lighting is always crucial to your work as a make-up artist. Lighting is the art of painting with light and shade; it can make a set look dull or interesting. The basics of lighting consist of a main light, the *key light*; a secondary light, the *fill light*, which has less intensity and can model or sculpt the subject; and a *back light*, which separates the subject from the background.

It is not only the *amount* of light that affects the subject, but also the *direction* from which it falls. *Cross-lighting* is the illumination of the actor, on the front of his face, from two directions at equal distance but opposite angles. Cross-lighting has the effect of emphasising wrinkles on the face and, whilst excellent for an ageing make-up, it is not flattering for a 'beauty' make-up.

In *film work* the exterior work on location is natural: that is, the sun acts as the key light. The secondary or fill light is provided by reflection or using arc lamps.

Television lighting is generally fixed on a set, with a scheme similar to that used for stage lighting. Each relies on overhead fill lighting and side key lighting, with floor fill lights to lessen the facial shadows.

Lighting for *video* is generally much flatter than for cinematography: less detail will be picked up, so the make-up needs to be stronger or much of the effect will be lost.

For *still camera* work an electronic flash is used when exposing the film. This produces a very intense and rapid flash of light. The 'freezing' action of electronic flash at high speed provides sharp-looking pictures. In commercial photography this is the most widely used method.

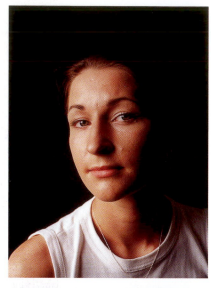

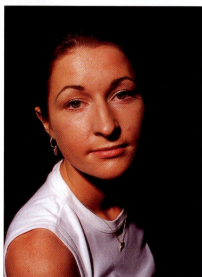

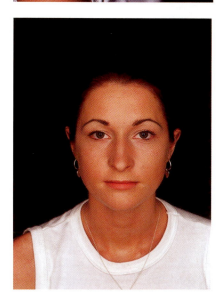

The effects of lighting

Effects of lighting on make-up can be practised with normal domestic lights.

1 Seat your model under an overhead light, suspended from the ceiling without a shade. Observe the unflattering shadows in the eye, nose and mouth areas.

2 Place a lamp to one side of your model. Observe the deep shadow on the side of the face that is not illuminated.

3 Put the lamp below your model's face. Note the grotesque effects of unnatural-looking shadows.

Effects of lighting on colour

Light can change colours dramatically, as when the colours drain away from a landscape if the sun is obscured by a dark cloud. A face is never the same colour over its entire surface: it will be darker in shadow areas and lighter where the light strikes the surface. This interplay of light and shade, and its effect on the colour of a facial feature, helps to define the features and reveal them as three-dimensional.

Activity – Drawing light and shade (2)

With some white cartridge paper and soft pencil, and using a fellow student as a model, draw a face, putting in the light and dark areas. (Photographs can be used, but a live model is best.) Keep to the full-face pose as this avoids the problems of foreshortening of the features that arise when the face is turned away from you.

The face must not be too brightly lit; the shadows cast would be very dense and consequently harsh, making the contrast between areas of light and shade too wide. Aim at a soft diffused light, with the light source to one side of the head. This is the most flattering light: it brings out the roundness of the head and the modelling of the features.

If the shadows still look too dark, you may be able to correct this with a little reflected light placed on the opposite side to the light source. This can be achieved using a white-painted board or other white material, positioning it so that some of the light is reflected back into the shadows. Alternatively, another light could be placed on this side.

Observe the shadows and the highlights which reveal the bone structure and the contours. Note that the areas of the face most likely to be in shadow are beneath and along the jaw and under the brows and cheeks (particularly if these are prominent). Other shaded areas are at the sides of the nose and immediately under it, especially in the depression running from the nose to the middle of the upper lip. There is usually a shadow just beneath the centre of the bottom lip, provided that the lip is fairly full. The highlighted areas are generally on top of the nose, across the forehead and on the fullest part of the cheeks.

Straight make-up

2

Introduction

Having studied the face and learnt something about facial anatomy, you can begin some basic make-up. The most fundamental technique here is known as **straight make-up**. Straight make-up may incorporate *corrective make-up* and **camouflage make-up**. It can overlap into beauty and fashion but its real function is to enhance, to correct and to define the person's face, rather than to change it. Straight make-up is applied to news announcers, politicians and other people being interviewed, in documentaries, modern-day dramas, soaps, comedies and light entertainment.

In general, straight make-up should be light and understated. Naturally, some women will prefer a heavier make-up and there are always exceptions to any rule. But make-up should never be perceptible on men and it is an art in itself to achieve a make-up look that doesn't look made-up!

Planning the make-up

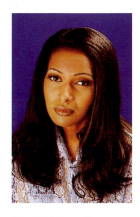

Straight make-up

Make-up should always be planned prior to application. Before starting a make-up, take into account the following checklist:

- **Suitability** Make-up must match the needs of the required image.
- **Choice of colours** The analysis must be made against a neutral colour and should take into account colours to be worn, eye colour and hair colour. The hair should be well off the face and secured, and the model's face should have been cleansed, toned and moisturised.
- **Skin care** You should check whether the model has any skin or eye allergies.
- **Timing** Assess the time needed to apply the make-up. Be realistic and negotiate as necessary with the other personnel involved.

Make-up for women

A professional straight make-up on a woman comprises the application of some or all of the following products, applied in this order.

1 Foundation (base)
- To establish the correct skin tone.
- To obscure any differences of colour in the face.
- To provide a 'canvas' on which to work.

2 Concealer or camouflage cream
- To take away shadows under the eyes, to disguise nose-to-mouth lines and to cover any blemishes not hidden by the foundation.

3 Powder (loose, translucent form)
- To fix the make-up base and to take away the shine.

4 Cheekcolour or blusher
- To provide colour in the cheeks and to define the cheekbones.

5 Eyeshadow
- To provide a frame to the eyes.
- To project and define the eyes.

6 Eyebrow colour
- To define the brows.

7 Eyeliner
- To define the eyes, by painting or drawing a line close to the eyelashes.

8 Mascara
- To colour and emphasise the eyelashes.

9 False eyelashes
- Sometimes (when in fashion) to add definition to the eyes.

10 Lipcolour
- To colour the lips.
- To define or redefine the shape of the lips.

Although it is not always necessary to apply all of these items, it is best to consider each area in this sequence.

Straight make-up application

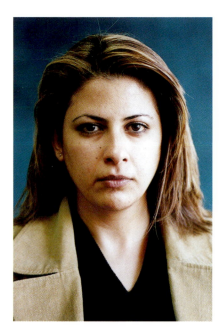
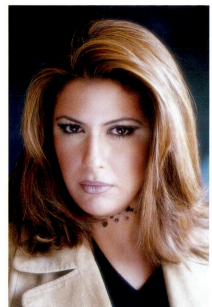

Before   After

Equipment and materials

General

- cleanser (milk or cream; unperfumed)
- toner (skin tonic – for example, rosewater with glycerine for dry skin, or rosewater with distilled witch hazel for greasy skin)
- moisturiser (unperfumed)
- tissues
- cottonwool
- cotton buds
- styptic pencil (for men's shaving cuts)
- cream or pads for removing eye make-up
- powder puffs
- sponges – natural, latex, or rubber stipple (according to requirements)
- gown
- headband

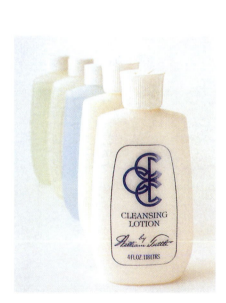

Skin-care products

Solvents

- brush cleaner
- nail-varnish remover

Eyelash accessories

- false eyelashes
- eyebrow tweezers
- eyelash curlers

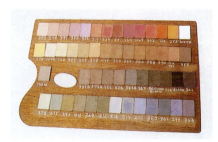

Blushers and eyeshadows

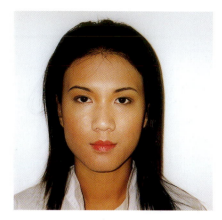

Straight make-up

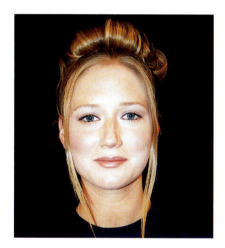

Straight make-up

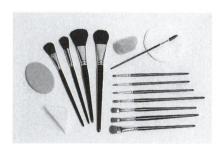

Brushes and sponges

Make-up

- foundations
- concealers
- loose powder
- blushers
- eyeliners
- mascara
- colour ranges for eyes
- lipsticks
- lipgloss

Brushes

- sable* domed brushes ($\frac{1}{4}$-inch and $\frac{1}{2}$-inch)
- sable* straight-topped brushes
- eyebrow brushes
- eyelash separators
- eyeliner brushes
- blusher brushes
- lip brushes
- powder brushes

*Ox, pony and goat brushes are much less expensive and are suitable for applying blusher and for brushing off powder, but they are too floppy to use when blending eyeshadow or grease or when highlighting or shading. Blending brushes *must* be sable.

Shaving equipment

- electric shaver
- wet razor and blades
- aftershave, gels or creams
- antiseptic ointment

Nail cosmetics

- cuticle-remover cream and sticks
- clippers
- buffers
- orange sticks
- assorted nail varnishes
- emery boards
- nail scissors
- nail repair glue
- false nails

Selecting the foundation

Foundations (or *bases*) are used to create a clear, healthy-looking complexion in the right colour. All blemishes and shadows should be painted out, yet the effect should be natural looking and not heavy in texture. The eyes, cheeks and lips should be made up to emphasise the best features of the face and to minimise the less desirable ones.

Selecting a shade of **foundation** to match someone's skin tone is the first step and the most important one. At first this will seem difficult, but with time and practice it will become automatic. The foundation should match the person's skin tone and be natural looking. At the same time it should provide an even film of colour and cover minor irregularities of skin tone such as redness. To test a foundation shade, place a tiny amount on the forehead. If the colour is correct, it will blend easily with the natural tone of the skin. This method of foundation selection is used by most make-up artists.

There is no need to have hundreds of different-coloured foundations. By using your eyes and developing your colour sense, you will learn to mix a colour for any skin type. The professional brands are the best to use. They are made especially for the media, are the right consistency and have a wider colour choice than those made for the general public and sold in chemists' shops and department stores.

Each person's skin tone is a combination of red, brown, white and yellow, mixed in various combinations. To learn how to match a foundation colour, start by mixing a small quantity of these colours together and make an exact match for your own skin tone. Then do the same for as many other people as you can. Soon you will get used to estimating the amount of yellow in someone's skin tone at a glance. For black skins you will need more red and yellow than for white ones, otherwise the foundation will appear grey and dull.

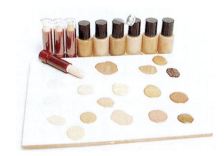

Liquid foundations and concealers

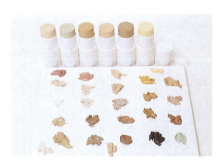

Panstiks

Types of foundations

- **Liquid foundations** Used for a natural look on young or clear skin, often for beauty work. They are applied using a damp sponge. There are many types and professional products tend to be the least sticky.

- **Cream foundations** Used for older skin or for greater coverage on younger skin. They should be used lightly.

- **Panstik foundations** Used for heavy coverage, as in theatre work. These greasepaints come in palettes and as sticks and have a greater density of pigment. Being greasy, they need powder to set them.

- **Camouflage foundations** Used for poor complexions and to cover scars, spots and blemishes (see page 46).

- **Pancake foundations** Used for body make-up and where a 'flat' look is required, as on bald heads. **Pancake** is normally too flat and dry for the face. It does not rub off on clothing, which makes it ideal for use on the body. It is also used for fantasy face painting. Pancakes are water-based foundations, applied using a wet sponge. They dry quickly to

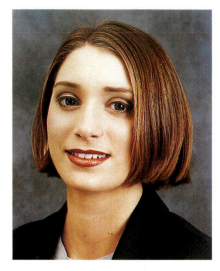

Straight make-up

Equipment and materials

- brushes (clean) in container
- cleanser, toner and moisturiser
- cottonwool and buds
- sponge and water in a small bowl
- foundations (assorted)
- loose powder
- concealers
- colour ranges for eyes
- blushers
- eyeliner and mascara
- eyebrow pencils
- tissues
- lip pencils
- lipsticks and lip gloss
- gown and headband
- powder puff

---

a matt finish and when dry can be buffed with a cloth to give a natural-looking sheen. Pancake is available in all colours as well as in skin tones.

- **Tint foundations** Used only on very clear skin or to enhance a tan. No powder is required. Tints can look good on men's skin.

Making up the face

Hygiene

- Always work cleanly and hygienically.
- Do not re-use brushes, sponges, powder puffs and the like. Keep them clean while in use, then wash them or throw them away. Throw away used cottonwool, tissues and cotton buds.
- Don't forget to put the lids back on jars and bottles when you've finished with them.

Preparation

1 Place a gown around the model.
2 Place tissues around the collar.
3 Put on the headband. At this point, study the face shape, features, skin tone and texture. Discuss preferences, ideas and colours.
4 Cleanse, tone and moisturise the skin. If the skin is dry, allow the moisturiser to sink in. If it is oily, blot the excessive grease using tissues. (A good skin preparation is essential for the smooth application of the make-up foundation.)
5 Choose a suitable base which matches the skin tone. Test this on the forehead as the light is particularly good on this area.

Applying the foundation

Having applied the moisturiser, you are now ready to apply the foundation.

1 With a barely damp sponge (natural or synthetic – try both types), apply a small amount of the foundation, starting on the forehead, working down the face, lightly and evenly across the eyelids, avoiding the mouth, blending under the chin, and onto the upper part of the neck.

Tip

Various tools can be used to apply foundation. A wedge, oval or round sponge may be best for a smoother or heavier base. A natural sponge, although not as smooth, may give a more natural look. Sometimes you will need to use your fingers, though this is less hygienic. You may find it convenient to cut a baby sponge into four pieces.

Tip

Loose powder can be sprinkled around the eyes, on top of cheekbones, to protect the base from 'spoiling' if any dark colours drop when applying eyeshadow powders. With a soft powder brush you can sweep the powder away afterwards.

However, take care when using compressed powders, whether eyeshadows or blushers. Use very little; you can always apply more. Use the tip of your brush for eyeshadows and test on the back of your hand first. Don't overload your brush. Leave no lines – blend the edges well.

Tip

Greys, browns, taupes and peaches are all good for a subtle natural look when applying eyeshadow.

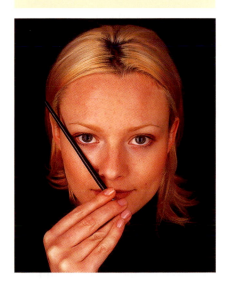

The nose-to-eye measuring technique

2 Use the clean side of the sponge to blend the edges away at the hairline on the forehead, around the ears and on the neck.

3 Use a clean brush to blend the foundation evenly around the sensitive eye areas, under the nose and around the nostrils.

Setting the foundation

1 To apply loose powder, dip the powder puff into the powder. Shake off any excess. Then tap the puff against the back of your hand, dislodging any remaining excess. There should not be too much powder on the puff at one time.

2 Roll the powder puff over the face, pressing firmly yet gently with a rocking motion, until the entire face is covered. More powder is usually needed down the centre part of the face. Don't forget the eyelids, under the chin and onto the neck. Be very sparing on the eye areas, especially below the eyes.

3 Brush off excess powder with a large soft **powder brush** for a smooth, even finish. Use the tip of the brush softly to avoid streaking the make-up.

Cheeks

To apply *blusher*, using a natural colour:

1 Feel for the top of the cheekbones. If necessary, ask the model to smile.

2 Apply blusher to the 'apple' of the cheek; brush upwards onto top of cheekbone. Use very little, simply to give the base colour some 'life'. More can be applied after working on the lips and eyes; by then you will be able to see the balance.

Eyes

To use subtle colours for a natural look on pale skin tones:

1 Lighten the brow bone with white *eyeshadow*, then with peach.

2 Apply taupe (pale grey-brown), starting at the outer edge of the eyelid and working towards the centre. Use grey to emphasise the outer edge.

3 When you are happy with the blending, apply the *eyeliner*. Use grey, brown or black. Keep this subtle. Begin at the start of the eyelash growth, but not too far into the inner corners of the eyes. Pull the eyelid taut gently with your fingertip and paint a thin line as close to the roots of the lashes as possible. If you want to blend the line, use a clean brush to do so.

4 The same method should be used along the bottom lashes. Do not draw a line further than the natural growth of lashes on the inside corner, nor further out on the outer corners than the outer edge of the eyebrow. Hold a pencil or brush to check on the distance.

Eyelashes

1 Apply *mascara* to the eyelashes on the lower eyelids using the tip of a brush. Stand behind the model. Hold the top lid up slightly and brush mascara through the eyelashes in downward strokes and then upwards on the underside of the lashes. Stand further around the model and repeat the procedure for the other eye. If you aren't using a proper make-up chair with a headrest, you can rest the model's head against your body.

2 Apply one or two coats of mascara, then brush through with a clean mascara comb or brush to separate the lashes and remove any excess blobs of mascara.

Eyebrows

1 Brush through.

2 Fill in any gaps or change the shape as required using: a suitable brush and powder; a pencil in short strokes; or, for a heavier look, paint on strokes with 'wet powder colour'.

3 At this point, define eye and cheek colour by adding more if necessary.

Tip

Powder eyeshadows are also good for applying to the eyebrows.

Lips

Lips are often the hardest part of the make-up. Precision is vital. Lips should be balanced out if there are any imperfections. Blotting, powdering and reapplying will make the lip colour last longer. Loose powder can be used on top of a glossy lipstick to make it more matt. For stability, you can rest your hand on a powder puff on the face, or rest your little finger on the chin. The edges should be drawn in first, then filled in.

1 Discuss the colour with the model (unless you are working to a brief).

2 *Lip pencil* can be used to define the shape first. With the *lipstick*, work from the corners up; or draw the top and bottom outline first, and then work from the corners up.

3 Lips can be evened out and enlarged; they can even be reduced if foundation is applied first. Work slowly but positively. Use the correct pressure. If you are too light you will tickle or irritate and it will be harder to create a line. If you press too hard you will move the lips. Ask the model to open and close her mouth as necessary.

4 Blot the lipstick and reapply it.

5 Check the make-up and powder again lightly, brushing off any excess with a large soft brush.

Lips

False eyelashes

From the natural look using individual lashes suitable for close-up on film to an exotic heavy-lashed look for the stage, **false eyelashes** can make an enormous difference to the eyes. For the best effect, however, they must be trimmed properly and attached as close to the real lashes of the eyes as possible.

The best – but most expensive – are made of real hair knotted onto a strip. Less expensive are the nylon ones, also in strip form. They are usually shaped, but tend to be too long for all but the largest eyes. Sometimes the eyelashes are available on long strips completely untrimmed – all the lashes are the same length.

Whatever the type of eyelashes, they should be individually fitted to the eyes and trimmed to suit the requirements of the make-up. The strip they are attached to should not be stuck too close to the inner corner of the eye, but further out where the eye curves upwards and the real eyelashes begin. The other end should finish at the place where the outer corner of the eye ends.

If the eyelashes are already shaped and you need to cut the strip, always cut the end where the lashes are shortest, so as not to lose the length of the outer lashes.

Equipment and materials

- eyelashes
- eyelash curlers
- eyelash adhesive
- eyelash tweezers
- fine brush
- cotton buds
- eyecolour (water-based)

Tip

Use a cotton bud to tap the eyelash into position.

Preparing the eyelashes

- To prepare the untrimmed type of eyelashes, cut them at an angle so that there is a left and a right lash, with the outer lashes about 12 mm in length and the inner ones 6 mm. Then cut every other hair about 3 mm shorter than the next, to give a feathered effect.

Applying the eyelashes

1. To apply the lashes, place the heavier, curved end on the outer part of the upper lashline, as close to the natural lashes as possible. Do not extend beyond the natural lash growth.

2. Some people use *eyelash tweezers* to place the strip in place, others prefer to use their fingers. The *eyelash adhesive* should be lightly stroked onto the underside of the strip before placing it gently on the eyelid.

3. When both sets of eyelashes have been correctly placed and the **adhesive** has dried, it will be necessary to go over the strip with eyeliner to disguise it. Taper the end of the painted eyeline with a fine, pointed brush to make the line look natural.

4. If the natural lashes are too straight it may be necessary to add mascara to attach them to the false ones. Another method is first to use *eyelash curlers* on the natural lashes, before applying the false ones.

5. Do not use pencil to line the eyelids as the grease in the pencil will cause the strip to become loose. Water-applied *eyeliner* is best. Always use a fine, pointed sable-hair brush.

6. For a wide-eyed look, you can attach one or two of the outer natural lashes to the corresponding false ones with eyelash adhesive. This works very well if the natural outer lashes are a bit 'droopy'.

Some false lashes are attached two or three hairs at a time. These are fixed into position by dipping each group of lashes into adhesive and placing them at the base of the natural lashes. They look effective when used at the outer corners only, or to replace a space in the natural lashline. The adhesive should be spread onto a plate or palette and a group of hairs should be held with tweezers and dipped into the adhesive so that the base is covered. Attach each group separately, in the direction of the natural curve of the lashes. The lashes can be trimmed to the length of the real lashes and coated with mascara as normal. The result will be undetectable in close-up. Individual lashes can be placed in the same way.

There are many varieties of false eyelashes, in varying densities of thickness and length. For strong effects, lashes are also available in gold, silver, red, blue, green and yellow; there are even multicoloured ones. Normally it is preferable to use brown lashes on fair-haired people and black ones on dark-haired people.

Equipment and materials

- cotton buds
- cleansing milk or eye make-up remover
- tissue

Removing the eyelashes

1   To remove the false eyelashes, take hold of the outer end of the strip with one finger, place a finger of the other hand on the centre of the closed eyelid, and gently peel off the strip.
2   Remove the bits of dried adhesive and wash off the mascara with a cotton bud soaked in cleansing milk or *eye make-up remover*. Place the lashes back in their box.
3   If the false lashes lose their curl, wind them round the curve of a pencil: roll a tissue around this and leave overnight. They should be curled again by the next morning.

Bottom lashes may be used when the top lashes are very heavy; they were much used in the 1960s. Bottom lashes can also be drawn in, using a fine brush and eyeliner; this is effective for opera, ballet and other stage work. Bottom lashes are not generally used in TV and film work today as they are not fashionable, but they are still used for some fantasy and light entertainment shows and, of course, in period or historical work where appropriate. Bottom lashes are applied in the same way as upper lashes.

Men

False eyelashes are not used on men. If a man has fair eyelashes it may be necessary to use mascara in order to define the eyes. Always apply sparingly and brush through afterwards with a clean brush to separate the eyelashes and remove excess mascara. In feature films or a long-running TV series it is better to tint a man's eyelashes, as tint will last for approximately six weeks.

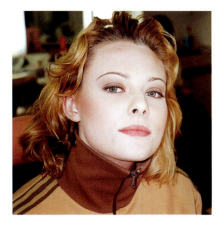

Sarah Jagger

Case Profile
Sarah Jagger, Make-up artist

How long have you been in the industry?
Eight months.

How did you get into it?
I took a three month Make-up Artist Course which provided me with valuable skills and an

understanding of what to expect within the industry. The 'starting out' process of freelance work can be very daunting, but I received so much professional support from my teachers and college that I was able to start building my CV and portfolio immediately. Whilst I was studying, I entered my portfolio of college work in the BBC Vision Brightest Sparks Competition and received a winning place. This gave me the opportunity to work on a children's television drama for five weeks and to exhibit my work and designs at the National Film Theatre.

What or who has been your most significant projects?

'Test Work' has been very significant to my career, as it helps me to use my own ideas and designs to establish a unique style in my portfolio.

What do you enjoy most about your work?

The design process – I love to take an idea from paper to a moving work of art. I also love the collaboration that needs to be done before the project can begin and the people you meet who invest their own creative ideas and experience.

And least?

The long hours can make you tired and separate you from your personal life when working on productions for long periods of time.

What advice would you give to people trying to get into this area of work now?

Be patient and determined. Even the most seemingly insignificant jobs can bring unexpected rewards.

A 1930s fashion look
Make-up artist Sarah Jagger

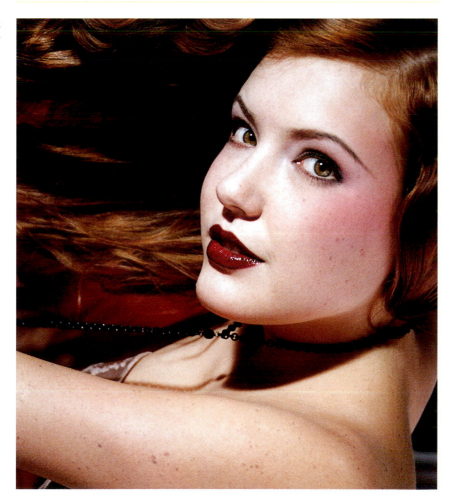

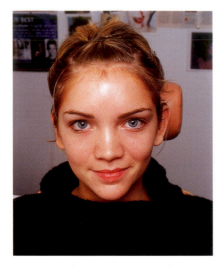

Before

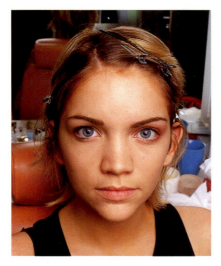

Foundation applied and eyeshadow on right eye

Activity – Step-by-step beauty make-up
(Make-up Artist: SARAH JAGGER. Model: LOUISA)

1. I applied laura mercier® foundation primer to the face followed by Clinique liquid sheer foundation.

2. I used concealer under the eyes and elsewhere to erase blemishes.

3. I set the foundation with yellow powder taking particular care under the eyes and around the nose.

4. I just brushed through the eyebrows to achieve a natural look.

5. I applied laura mercier® cream blush in Nutmeg on the eyelids, and blended it lightly up towards the eyebrows.

6. I applied brown/black eye shadow to the top eyelids, close to the lashes, blending into the eye socket creases, and under outer corners of the eyes.

7. I used pale shimmer cream on the lips and inner corners of eyes.

8. I applied black mascara – one coat only for natural effect – to the lashes, and then curled them with eyelash curlers.

9. I used cream blusher on the cheeks, blending towards the ears.

10. Pale shimmer was stippled on the upper cheek bones, and left unblended to provide maximum highlight effect for photograph.

11. Rather than use lipstick, for a natural effect foundation mixed with vaseline was placed on the centre of bottom lip.

12. Random pieces of hair were straightened and John Frieda sheer blonde® 'Funky Chunky' texturiser run through the hair to separate the layers and provide holding power.

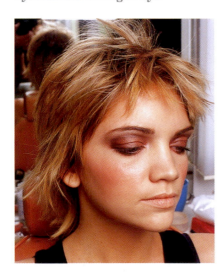

Dark cream eyeshadow and cream blusher on cheeks

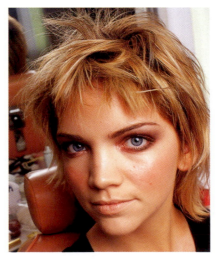

Shimmer added on upper cheekbones and around inner eye area

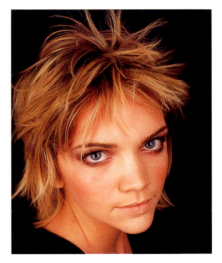

The finished look

Miscellaneous tips

Manner

- **To give confidence** Always work gently and calmly, with a friendly and relaxed manner.

General

- **To make the best use of make-up** For the maximum effect, use the minimum make-up. Apply it only when it is really needed, for example, there is often no need for an overall foundation.

Features

- **To emphasise the natural structure of the face** Use shading, both medium and light. Highlight prominent areas, such as the forehead, cheekbones and the shadows under the eyes. Warm the eyebrow bones by applying a light-coloured blusher. Highlight the top of the cheekbones.
- **To project a feature forward, or to diminish it** Reverse the natural shadows.

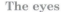 The eyes

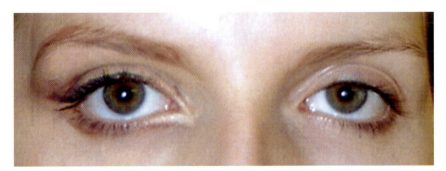

The eyes

- **To bring the eyes closer together** Put a darker colour on the eyelids, in the inner corners of the eyes.
- **To bring deep-set eyes 'out'** Lighten the socket line.
- **To 'lift' the outside of the eye** Shade the outside of the eye corner towards the eyebrow. Blend the shading away to nothing.
- **To 'lift' the eye** Apply a little eyelash adhesive to a couple of the outer corner eyelashes and attach these to the outer eyelid.
- **To disguise stubborn shadows under the eyes** Try applying a small circle of blusher to high cheekbones, in line with the centre of the eye: this will often distract the observer's eye from the shadows.

Age

Remember: the older the person, the lighter should be both the make-up application and the colours.

- **To avoid 'ageing' the model** Don't apply too much foundation or eye make-up. Don't use too much foundation or powder in creases and laughter lines. Don't emphasise lines going downwards. Don't light eyebag areas.

Make-up for men

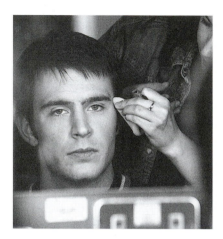

A straight make-up on actor Jack Davenport in *The Cookie Man*. Make-up artist Leda Shawyer

The make-up for a man should be natural-looking, yet at the same time corrective and flattering. It should be subtle enough not to appear made-up to the general public and yet should improve his image for TV cameras and newspaper photographers.

Do not apply a base all over a man's face unless he is particularly pale or grey looking. If it is necessary to change his skin tone, use a liquid foundation lightly, as a wash of colour, so that it is almost transparent.

The most important details to bear in mind are the shadows under the eyes and the beardline. If the latter looks too dark, it should be lightened with a pinkish, yellow or orange colour, which will neutralise and 'kill' the blueness of the beard shadow. This is necessary only on dark-haired men whose beardlines show a prominent 'six o'clock shadow'.

Grey hairs and bald or thinning patches can be darkened with make-up. Under heavy studio lights, bald heads should be made up so that they do not shine too much. Use a pancake or liquid body make-up, not grease-based products, to give a matt appearance.

If a make-up base has been applied to the face, don't forget to darken the backs of the hands with pancake. Avoid using grease or cream make-up on the hands. Even after powdering, this would come off on the clothes. The ears too should be made up as on camera they often appear too red. Be careful not to blend the face make-up too far down the man's neck as it could stain his shirt collar. Tuck a paper tissue around the neck collar whilst working under the chin and onto the neck. Hair should be tidied with a comb or brush in the normal way. Make sure there are no stray hairs sticking out: the outline should be tidy. Hairspray, wax, gel or grease may also be used. Usually though it is best to leave the hair looking natural, especially on an older man who is not used to using hair preparations. If the make-up is for an interview to take place outdoors, then spraying the hair is not a good idea.

The beardline

Toning down a beardline

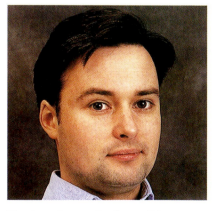

Toning down the beardline
Before

1   Apply a foundation, very lightly.
2   Don't remove shadows unless these are really bad; to do so tends to make the face look too feminine. A little lightening under heavy eyebags is usually enough.

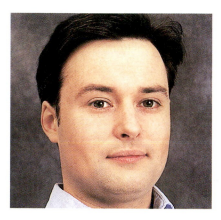

After

Equipment and materials

- foundation
- camouflage cream
- stipple brush
- powder and brush
- natural sponge
- cottonwool
- stipple sponge
- eyeliner (water-based)
- mascara

3 Tone down the beard using a camouflage cream applied lightly by means of a rubber *stipple sponge*. Apply a foundation on top of this. For a very heavy beard shadow, an orange camouflage can be used to take away the blue. This works particularly well on Indians or men with black hair.

4 Never use blusher on a man. If colour is needed in the cheeks, apply a brown or tan colour using a *natural sponge* with a stippling movement.

5 Powder lightly and brush off any excess with a clean powder brush. To remove the powdered look, press damp cottonwool on the cheeks and the nose area. This also helps the make-up to last longer under hot lights.

6 When standing by on the set, apply more powder only if the model's face is shining too much. If asked by the cameraman to apply more powder, don't forget to brush off the excess with a clean brush so that it doesn't look obvious.

Filling in or changing a beardline

1 Apply a bluish-black colour. Black is too hard so it is better to mix blue and dark brown from your palette. Use very little and stipple it on using a natural sponge. A special stipple sponge may be used as well as a natural one.

2 Remember that a beardline will make the man look older.

3 If the eyes 'disappear', use eyeliner. Apply it in dots between the lashes – never paint a heavy line on a man. Use a water-based liner and tone this down with water. Use brown or grey on fair-haired men and dark brown on dark-haired men.

4 Mascara can be used on freckly, sandy-haired pale faces, but don't use much and brush it through the lashes carefully. Use shades of brown, never black.

Corrective make-up

The use of colour

A 'straight' make-up may not be sufficient to hide defects such as scars, shadows under the eyes and minor skin blemishes. In such cases it may also be necessary to use colour to conceal a defect. *Concealing colours (concealers)* are available ready-made, or you can mix your own on a palette.

- **Too much red in the skin tone** Use yellow concealer before or after applying the foundation. In extreme cases of redness, green can be used to tone down the colour, but this should be used with caution. Green can take away so much colour that it makes the person look ill.

Skin discolouration

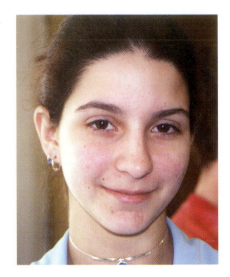 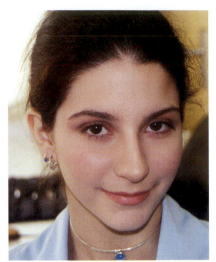

Before   After

- **A blue-black beardline** Blue can be counteracted by applying orange, for example to tone down the beardline on a man with six o'clock shadow.
- **Blue-black shadows under the eyes** Orange works well in hiding these, on skin tones ranging from olive to black. For dark shadows under the eyes on pale-skinned people, use either the matching skin tone or, if the shadow looks grey, add some pink to the area with a touch of Veil Rose to lift the colour.

Hiding shadow under the eyes
with orange

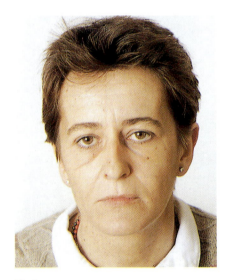 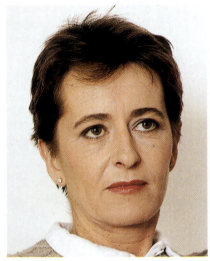

Before   After

- **Grey shadows** Pink will take these away on pale skin tones.

Most make-up artists apply the corrective concealing colour before using a foundation, but it can also be applied afterwards.

Highlighting and shading

The term 'corrective make-up' also includes the use of highlighting and shading, perhaps the most important skills in the make-up artist's repertoire.

Highlighting is the blending of a shade lighter than the foundation in order to make a feature more obvious. This might be used, for example, to bring out deep-set eyes or a weak chin. *Shading* is the blending of a shade darker than the foundation in order to diminish a feature. A large nose could be shaded at the sides to make it appear thinner, for instance, or a double chin could be made less obvious by shading.

In straight and beauty make-up, highlighting and shading are often referred to as *contouring*. The process can enhance a good bone structure or, if the face is plump, give the illusion of one.

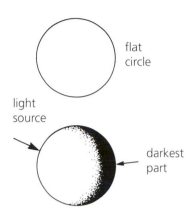

flat circle

light source

darkest part

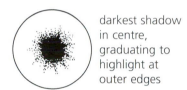

darkest shadow in centre, graduating to highlight at outer edges

Using light and shade to make a flat circle look round

Principles of light and shade

If you draw a round circle on a piece of paper, it will appear flat. To make it appear rounded you need to add some shadow and highlighting. By placing some dark shading around the outer circle of the 'ball' and by blending this shadow to nothing, leaving a white highlight, you can make the circle look like a white ball.

If you draw a similar circle and this time add a strong colour in the centre, blending this outwards to a highlight at the outer edges, the circle will again look like a ball. This process is similar to the technique used in blending cheek colour.

 Activity – Drawing light and shade (1)

1 Throw a piece of drapery across the back of a chair near a source of light such as a window or a side lamp.

2 Study the light and shade in the folds of the cloth. The brightest parts will have light shining directly onto them. The darkest areas will be those where the light does not reach.

3 Using a soft pencil, draw onto plain white paper the drapery as you see it. Draw the outline first, then fill in the details of the folds, softly smudging the edges of the shading. Try to make the folds of the cloth look rounded.

The object of this exercise is to improve your drawing skills, to develop your sense of observation and to help you become aware of the effect of light on any object. The light from the window creates 'highlights' on the folds of the cloth. The darkest, shadowed areas are furthest away from the source of light. The graduation of intensity makes the folds of cloth look rounded.

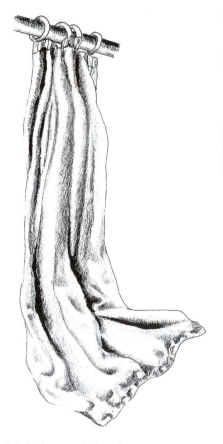

Lighting and shading

Applying these principles to make-up

Assessing what is needed

To begin the make-up, ask your model to tuck her chin down, and at the same time to look up into the mirror without raising her head. Most people will have dark circles under their eyes. On younger faces the shadows will be slight, although even children may have dark circles, either through lack of sleep or by reason of inheritance within their family.

On closer examination you will notice that there is a shadow running from the nose to the corners of the mouth. Apart from this the face may have blemishes, or patches of redness. After the foundation has been put on, you can mix a skin tone somewhat lighter than the overall colour and use this to paint in the circles under the eyes, covering any blemishes with a small brush. Blend the edges carefully. Redness can be toned down by adding more yellow to the concealing colour. (Concealing is not the same as highlighting, though both use a colour lighter than the base tone. The concealing colour should hide and tone in with the rest of the face tone, whereas a highlighting colour is to draw attention and to emphasise a particular feature.)

In certain contexts the performer is presumed already to be perfect for the part: the make-up is simply to make him or her as attractive as possible. This applies to the many people who appear on television but who are not actors, such as weather forecasters, interviewers and interviewees. Only slight adjustments may be necessary, such as shortening the nose, darkening the eyebrows, or reducing a dark beardline and covering blemishes.

Adjusting the structure of the face

Earlier on, when you were sketching a face on paper, you learned that the ideal face can be divided horizontally: from the hairline to the eyes; from the eyes to the bottom of the nose; and from the bottom of the nose to the tip of the chin. When the balance is not ideal, make-up can be used to improve it.

- **If the forehead is too high** Darken the forehead around the hairline with a colour two shades darker than the base colour. The colour must be blended downwards so that it gradually disappears into the foundation.

- **If the forehead is too low** Follow the same principle, but this time you will apply a colour two shades lighter than the foundation. Paint it close to the hairline in a wide equal band. As before, blend it downwards so that there is no line of demarcation.

- **If the forehead is too narrow or too wide** Add shadows or highlights at the outer sides, near the temples. Be careful not to shade in the temple areas too much, however. As you know from your previous 'skull' make-up, if overdone the effect will be ageing.

- **If the chin is too long** Shade the lower part.

Tip

Look in the mirror frequently and turn your model's head to observe it from the side view. If you are right-handed, always stand on the right-hand side when you work (and vice versa if you are left-handed).

You may find it easier to blend shading down the sides of the face with a damp sponge – but apply the line under the cheekbones with a brush. Check that the shading on both sides is equal, or the face will appear lopsided.

Now apply highlights to the tops of the cheekbones, carefully blending these away at the edges.

- **If the chin is too short** Highlight the lower part.
- **If the face is too flat or too round** Shading under the cheekbones is a classic aid to beauty and can make a flat or round face look more interesting.

When *drawing* you can blend edges with your fingers; when painting people's *faces*, however, it is both easier and more hygienic to use good-quality sable-haired brushes.

Remember: when selecting a colour for *shading*, use a liquid or cream two shades darker, but in the same tone as the natural skin colour; when *highlighting*, select one that is two shades lighter.

 Activity – Lighting and shading in make-up

Try some lighting and shading on one another's faces. Try to make them look rounder or longer. Use very little make-up, the more subtle the better. It must not look painted on, but should seem like natural shadows and highlights.

 Activity – Making up a face **Time: 1 hour**

Choose a type of make-up that involves the use of light and shade to create the required effect. It can be a 'beauty' make-up or one that makes your model look fatter or thinner. The idea is to choose a make-up that gives you practice in modelling with colour, either to flatter the person's face or to achieve the opposite.

1 First study the face, then decide what to do. Draw a sketch or chart and make written notes of what you are going to do to achieve the result. Where will you put the shading? Where will you put the highlights?

2 Choose and assemble your materials. Lay them out neatly on your working space, putting clean water in a bowl and having everything ready to hand.

3 Wash your hands.

4 Place a wrap around your model to protect her clothes and a hairband to keep the hair off her face.

5 Clean and moisturise her face. Test the skin for colours.

6 Apply the make-up.

7 Throughout the make-up, keep checking in the mirror to view the result and to check that the blending is balanced on either side of the face.

8 When you look in the mirror, check that the shading and lighting are not too heavy, that the colours are harmonious and suit your model's skin.

9 Now throw away all the used cottonwool, cotton buds and tissues. Pour a little brush cleaner into a small bowl. Clean your brushes and wipe them with a tissue. Put the bottle of brush cleaner away again. Put the tops back on all of the containers.

10 If you are working in a group, seek your tutor's appraisal. It is a good idea also to look at other students' make-ups, as much can be learned from constructive criticism and praise.

11 Take photographs for your own reference later.

12 Finally, remove your model's make-up.

Make-up chart

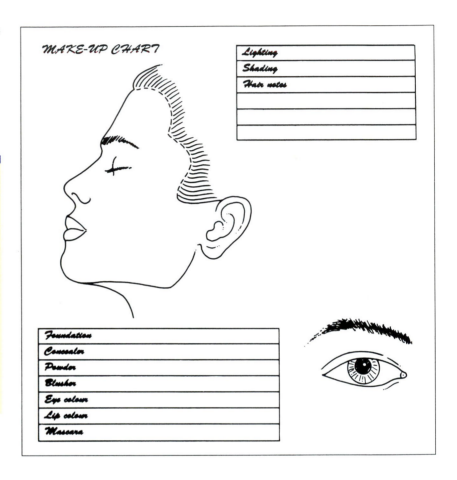

Tip

Whilst applying the make-up, be considerate towards your model. Don't lean on her head with your hand. Don't jerk her head around when looking in the mirror. If required, ask her politely to turn her head to a different angle. If applying lipstick, it may help to rest your hand on a powder puff placed on her chin.

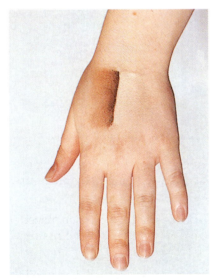

Blending

Blending

Blending means graduating the intensity of a colour – whether a darker colour for shading, or a lighter one for highlighting. The technique of graduating a colour from its strongest tone to its lightest, until it disappears into the skin tone, is one used constantly in every area of make-up.

 Activity – Blending

Practise blending by applying a line of make-up on the back of your hand. Using a sable brush, a cosmetic sponge or your fingertips, gradually reduce the amount of colour from the darkest point to the lightest (downwards), until the final edge fades into the skin.

Corrective make-up, showing
uses of lighting and shading

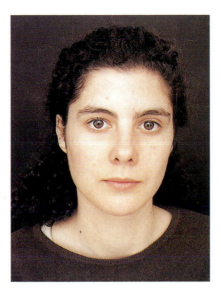

Before

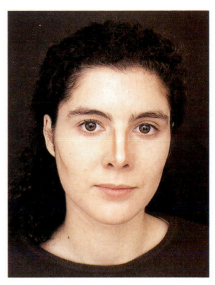

Slimming the nose

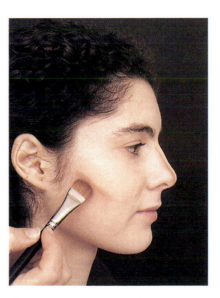

Slimming the side of the face

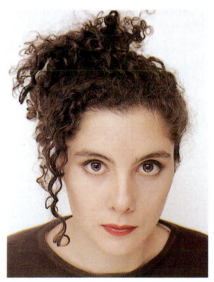

Finished effects

Body make-up

Make sure that all areas of the skin which may show on camera are made up to blend in with the face. Pancake or liquid body make-up should be used, in the same shade as the face make-up.

Men's ears in particular are apt to look very red if a light is placed behind them. Hands will look paler unless made up. (When making up the hands, do the backs only – not the palms.)

If there isn't time to apply body make-up, make sure that the facial skin tone matches other exposed parts of the body.

Body make-up

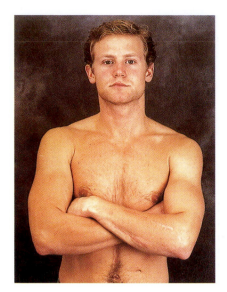 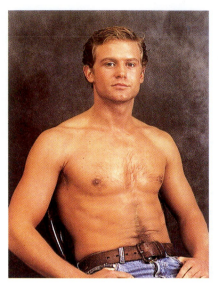

Before: the facial skin tone is uneven and the body too pale; there are also very obvious scars on the stomach and arms

After: the face and body tone have been evened out with water-based body make-up. The scars have been made less prominent with camouflage make-up

Removing the make-up

When the actor has finished filming, the director will release him or her and the make-up artist must remove the make-up. With character or special effects make-up, this can be time consuming and may involve the use of special solvents. With straight corrective make-up the procedure is simpler and merely involves cleansing, toning and moisturising.

An unperfumed simple *cleansing milk* or *cream* should be massaged onto the face and then wiped with *tissues* or *cottonwool*. Cottonwool soaked in warm water and squeezed until damp is good for cleansing the face efficiently. On men's faces it is better to use tissues, as cottonwool often sticks to their beardline. Some male actors prefer using *baby wipes*.

Toner should be applied after cleansing, to remove traces of grease. *Moisturiser* can then be applied to the face (especially on women). Many men prefer simply to wash their faces with soap and water; make sure you have a clean *towel* available.

Time spent on the make-up

How much time should be spent on each make-up?

Time is valuable, if the *shooting schedule* is not to be held up. Ensure that you work effectively to meet *deadlines*.

How long each make-up will take must be considered carefully; a *test make-up* will determine how long you need. Liaison is essential between the costume, make-up and hair departments. The assistant director (AD) will arrange the actors' transport and arrival in the mornings and will ask how long to allow for costume, make-up and hair.

The amount of time needed to complete a make-up is often difficult to determine. Each make-up is an original design and the problems involved are variable, depending on its complexity.

A rough guide

- **Straight corrective make-up, with tidy hair: man** 15 minutes.
- **Straight corrective make-up, with tidy hair: woman** 15 minutes.
- **Beauty make-up and hair: man** 30 minutes.
- **Beauty make-up and hair: woman** 1 hour 30 minutes.
- **Period make-up and hair using facial hair: man** 1 hour.
- **Period make-up and hair using wig: woman** 1 hour 30 minutes.
- **Fantasy make-up using wig: man** 1 hour.
- **Fantasy make-up using wig: woman** 1 hour 30 minutes.
- **Black eye, bruise, simple cut** 15 minutes.
- **Ageing make-up using bald cap, wig and old-age stipple** 1 hour 30 minutes.
- **Ageing make-up using bald cap and prosthetics** 2–3 hours.

Role of the make-up artist working in skin camouflage

Camouflage make-up creams are mainly used in hospitals and clinics throughout the world for the purpose of normalising the appearance of people suffering from any form of skin disfigurement. The patients needing this remedial treatment, through reasons of birth, accident or disease, are often referred to the make-up artist after undergoing plastic surgery. They are usually distressed by some aspect of their appearance and the make-up artist has to provide the technical skills of hiding the disfigurement and to teach them how to do it themselves in the simplest way possible. By doing this skilfully, the make-up artist contributes to the patient's confidence and self-esteem.

Because of the nature of the task it is vital that the make-up consultant builds up a trust with the person (who could be a man, woman or child) and has a tactful, sympathetic and professional manner. This is not an area of work where the make-up artist can

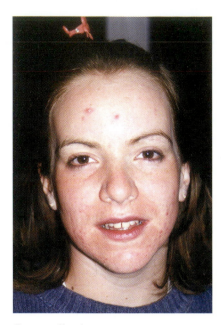

**Camouflaging acne
Before**

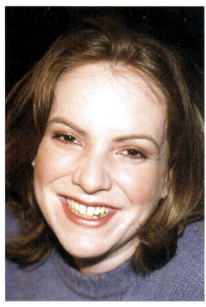

After

show feelings of pity or revulsion. For this reason the make-up consultants tend to be nurses who have attended a camouflage make-up course. Many hospitals, particularly those with burns and cancer units, have a camouflage service to show patients how to apply the specialised creams on skin areas that benefit from being camouflaged.

A knowledge of normal corrective and fashion make-up is a great advantage to camouflage artists, as it is all part of improving the person's appearance. For example, if a woman has an area around the mouth, chin or neck which needs camouflage work, it is a good idea also to show her how to enhance her eyes with normal cosmetics, thus drawing attention away from the affected area. When treating men and children, this is not possible because they need to look completely unmade up, so it is enough simply to cover the affected areas.

It is always very important to work out the simplest, easiest way for men and children or they will be discouraged from doing it for themselves. If several shades of camouflage creams are needed to match the skin tone, then the make-up consultant should mix the right blend of colours and re-pot it for the patient. Women are generally used to applying cosmetics. After the camouflage cream has been applied they are able to carry on doing their make-up in the usual way.

Skin camouflage work requires a special type of person to interact with patients who have had major cancer and burn operations. Nurses are usually best suited to this type of work, provided they can learn the technical skills of applying the make-up. However, there are also professional make-up artists who do well in this field, working in many clinics, particularly plastic surgery units. There is also work available camouflaging skin disorders or scarring due to birthmarks, vitiligo, road traffic victims, surface thread veins, dog bites, acne, eczema, small burns, tribal markings and tattoos.

For the make-up artist working in print and entertainment, camouflage skills have their place in hiding any blemishes which cannot be effectively covered by consumer fashion ranges. The usual problems faced by make-up artists include dark circles under the eyes, bruises, tattoos, spots, nervous rashes, cold sores, shaving rashes, cuts and very dark beardlines.

Camouflage products

Camouflage products differ from ordinary cosmetics in that they have greater covering qualities, are resistant to the harmful rays of the sun and are waterproof. They also have a far greater variety of colours for all ethnic skin tones.

Their holding power is better than fashion products, designed to stay in place whilst leading a normal active life. They are also easy to apply and simple to remove. There are five ranges of camouflage products available in single pots for individual use and palettes for professional use containing small amounts of all the colours.

Veil cover cream is produced by Thomas Blake & Company, UK

An excellent cream with a fine ointment base. The basic colours are called Medium, Dark, Suntan, Natural Medium, Tan, Natural Tan, Peach and White, plus several dark browns, Yellow, Green, Mauve and Rose. The creams are light in texture and suitable for small blemishes and where a very light cover is needed. It is the most useful range for make-up artists working in film, TV, fashion and theatre since it does not give a mask-like effect. It is the best Caucasian skin tone range, brilliant for light-coloured skin tones. The packaging is flimsy in order to keep the costs down, so it is best for make-up artists to transfer the colours to an empty paintbox, which provides easier transportation.

Dermacolor is produced by Kryolan, Germany

The Dermacolor camouflage system is very well known amongst make-up artists because Kryolan produces a whole range of professional products from beauty to special effects made specifically for use in television, feature films and theatre.

The Dermacolor range has 24 shades of cover creme contained in a strong metal paintbox, and also plastic containers with smaller amounts of the products that are lighter to carry around in a kit box. Whilst the colours range from very light to dark, they have very good colours for rich, dark skin tones. The lighter shades of creamy yellow are great for Asian skins.

Keromask is produced by Christy Cosmetics

A greasier consistency than all the other ranges, so suitable for very dry skins. Because of its more liquid texture it comes packaged in tubes as well as pots. The range has good coverage and choice of colours, but because of its greasy texture is not widely used by make-up artists. However, it is used extensively in hospitals and clinics, particularly in burns units where the patients' skin texture may be very dry. Keromask is also useful for mixing with other brands for a texture with more lubrication.

Covermark, USA

Covermark cremes are another useful range of camouflage products used in hospitals and clinics that are quite heavy in texture, so have a good coverage. Colours are similar to the other brands ranging from light to dark and made to be mixed together to obtain the exact shade of colour required.

Dermablend Corrective Cosmetics, Flori Roberts, USA

Dermablend has 15 shades of cover cremes ranging from ivory to the darkest ebony. These also have good coverage. Whilst suitable for all skin tones, they are particularly useful for the warm golden browns necessary for dark skins.

Camouflage powders

All the companies that produce camouflage cremes also make a loose powder for *setting* the colours. The powder is unperfumed and transparent to avoid changing the colour of the cream. Sometimes it is a fine white talc. Baby talcum powder can also be used. All the colours in the different brands may be mixed with one another to obtain the required shade and texture.

Some of the cremes are for a specific purpose, for example, the mauve is for counteracting harsh orange lighting, the green to tone down extreme redness and the bluish/grey colour is for filling in men's beardlines.

All the ranges have a very natural looking blusher when adding warmth for a pinker tone and the bright yellow is good for mixing with pale skin tone shades for a sun-tan effect.

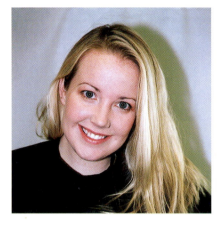

Shauna O'Toole

Case Profile
Shauna O'Toole, Make-up artist

When and how did you start in the business?
The day I met my friend's mum, who was a successful make-up artist in both film and TV, I realised that the art of make-up application could become a career. From that point I volunteered to help in my university theatre productions and the Colorado Opera tours. I fell in love with the atmosphere and the art.

Was there a turning point in your career?
Absolutely. On my second job, the make-up artists were not team players and I observed how their bad attitudes created a domino effect. Their negativity became contagious and the production nearly collapsed. I realised not to take it personally. Cinematic make-up takes true teamwork and negative people are everywhere. It's up to us as individuals in this business to roll with the punches and make the best of the situation.

What do you think are important qualities for a make-up artist?
A positive attitude. A career as a make-up artist is based primarily on human interaction and a positive attitude attracts clientele.

How has your career changed your life?
After studying business and marketing at university, I worked for an advertising firm for a year but realised that I wasn't happy. This is when I decided to hop on a plane to London and take a year long course at the Delamar Academy. I haven't looked back since. Has my life changed? Oh yes, I'm much happier because I'm making money doing something I love.

What have been your most satisfying moments?
The moments I step back and I appreciate the work I have done. I have no regrets as the mistakes I've made in the business have only made me a better make-up artist.

I'll never know too much and I look forward to the many things I have yet to learn.

What advice would you offer to young people entering the industry?
Have a positive attitude, work hard and be determined. No matter how much talent you have, if you have a bad attitude you should opt for an alternative career. Don't give up! If you prove yourself people will notice and doors will open miraculously from nowhere. Love your line of work and the money seems to follow.

Do you think the film industry is glamorous?
No, not at all. I think many make-up artists decide they want to join the profession in order to mingle with famous actors and dine with the rich and famous, but this isn't realistic. Being a professional make-up artist is the furthest thing from glamorous as it is your duty to focus on the actor or model, not on yourself.

What do you consider to be the best and worst aspects of being a make-up artist?
The best aspects are the creative environment and the teamwork. The worst aspect is the entertainment industry's fickle job market. However, it's worth the wait for a great job.

Skin tones

Camouflaging acne

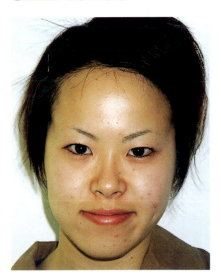 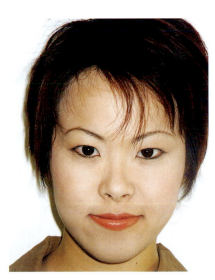

Before   After

It is difficult to define particular skin colouring since nearly everyone nowadays is a mixture of different ethnic mixes across the world. Our skin tones are due to intermarriages, lifestyle and the climates of the countries we live in. The following guide is based on the country of origin and may be used for reference because, as a student, it is necessary to start somewhere, though experience and practice are the best learning methods. The guide lists skin tones from the palest to the darkest with countries of origin and shades of camouflage creams that might be useful for mixing to find the exact match to the skin.

Countries of origin	*Camouflage creams*
Norway, Sweden, Denmark, Finland, Canada, North America, Western Europe, New Zealand, Australia	Veil: Natural, Medium, Natural Medium Tan, White, Peach Dermacolour: D0, D1, D2, D3, D6, D7 Covermark: Peach, Light White, Medium Keromask: No. 9 (light), No. 2 (white) Dermablend: Chroma 1, Chroma 2
India, Pakistan, Bangladesh, East Europe, West Europe, Canada, Middle East	Veil: White, Dark, Natural Tan, Tan Dermacolour: D0, D3, D4, D5, D6, D7, D8 Covermark: White, Medium Brunette, Rose Brown Keromask: No. 1 (brown), No. 10 (medium), No. 2 (white) Dermablend: Chroma No. 2, 2A, 3
China, Japan, Middle East, Bangladesh, Pakistan, Northern India	Veil: White, Dark, Suntan, Dark No. 2, Dark No. 3 Dermacolour: D0, D4, D5, D8, D9, D10, D18, D19 Covermark: White, Rose Dark, Dark Brown Keromask: No. 2 (white), No. 1 (brown), No. 10 (medium), No. 11 (dark), No. 7 (chestnut), No. 5 (yellow) Dermablend: Chroma No. 2, 2A, 3
Zimbabwe, Caribbean, Nigeria, Uganda, North American Indian, Southern India, Sri Lanka, Congo, Malawi, Zaire, Bangladesh, Japan, Middle East	Veil: Dark No. 2, Dark No. 3, Brown Dermacolour: D4, D5, D6, D8, D9, D10, D11, D13, D18, D19, D20 Covermark: No. 1 Keromask: No. 11 (dark), No. 5 (yellow), No. 7 (chestnut) Dermablend: Chroma No. 6, No. 7
Uganda, Sudan, Zimbabwe, Tanzania, Zambia, Malawi, Zaire, Mozambique	Dermacolour: D15, D16, D17, D40 Keromask: No. 7 (chestnut), No. 8 (umber), No. 4 (rose), No. 6 (black)

Orange

Dermacolour has a bright orange, which is useful for applying to dark shadows under the eyes on people from India and Pakistan. The orange will take away the blue-black appearance of the shadow without making it look grey. The same orange can be stippled lightly over a heavy beardline on men with very dark skin tones.

The basic kit

- camouflage palettes
- cleansing cream, rosewater, witch hazel for cleansing and removing grease on the skin
- cottonwool
- natural sponges
- stipple sponges
- camouflage own brand powder or unscented talcum powder
- cream rouge (Veil rose, Dermacolour D32 or Covermask rouge)

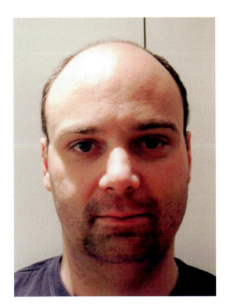

**Toning down a beardline
Before**

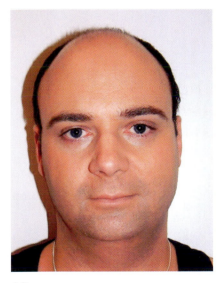

After

- sable make-up brushes, different sizes, soft powder brush
- cotton buds
- orange sticks or wooden spatulas
- scissors
- eyebrow tweezers
- normal make-up such as lipsticks, blushers, eyeliners, mascaras, eye shadows, eyelashes (natural daytime)

Matching the colour

Although there are a wide range of colours and many manufacturers of camouflage creams, sometimes an exact colour match will not be possible. Sometimes a person's skin tone may be halfway between two shades of cream. It is then easy to mix two equal amounts from the two creams to find the perfect colour match. When no exact match is available, the knowledge and experience of mixing colours is very important. The different ranges of creams react differently on people's skins, so the more variety of creams tested, the quicker you gain experience in achieving good results. To begin with you need to find the underlying skin tone, ignoring colours produced by blood being close to the skin surface, such as highly coloured cheeks. For example, someone with very pale skin of Celtic origin might have pink cheeks and freckles. To find such a pale colour you could try mixing Veil Medium (which has no pink in it), with Veil Tan (which has no yellow in it). For people from Libya with a dark skin tone, you could try Dermacolour D15, Dermacolour D16, or a mixture of the two colours. If that doesn't work, try mixing Covermark No. 8 and Covermark No. 3 or Keromask Chestnut No. 7 and Umber No. 8.

Countries close to the equator have an underlying skin tone which contains orange or red. This is why you sometimes get a greyish, ashen look, even when you think you have found the right colour. You can sometimes correct this by adding a little Keromask Rose to the colour before setting it with powder.

People from Middle Eastern countries often need Covermark No. 1, Covermark No. 8 or Keromask No. 7 (chestnut).

Everyone must be assessed individually. For testing the colours use a tiny amount on the skin you are working on and wait to see how the colour reacts.

Applying the colours

The skin must be clean and grease free, so for this reason there should be no moisturiser. The creams should be applied very thinly and sparingly so that the effect is natural and does not rub off. If one thin coat is not enough to obliterate the area you are trying to hide, you should powder the first coat lightly with a powder puff or cottonwool, brush off the excess powder with a soft brush and then blot the area gently with damp cottonwool. This removes any powder and sets the camouflage efficiently. If one layer of colour is

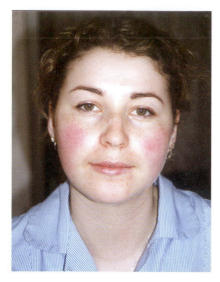

**Skin discolouration
Before**

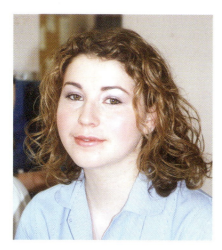

After

not enough, you can repeat the whole procedure several times in the areas where the blemish is still visible.

Sometimes an additional cream needs to be applied to the skin to change the shade slightly in order to tone in with the surrounding skin. An example of this might be when putting pink onto a cheek to copy the flushed colour on the other side of the face. This should be done before setting the area with powder, and damp cottonwool.

Tools used for applying colours

For tiny areas such as scars a small brush is more accurate. Small natural sponges are good for giving a natural effect. The sponge should be made wet to soften it, then squeezed out until it is just damp. Place the required colour in the palm of your hand and press the sponge against the colour to load it. Before using on the person's skin, first press it on the back of your hand to test the strength of colour. The natural sponge method provides a natural looking effect, which will tone down a blemish such as rosacea, while allowing some of the original colour to show through. This often looks better than a dense, mask-like look.

Covering a tattoo

Most make-up artists have to cover tattoos at some time. The easiest method is first to use a colour on the darkest part of the tattoo which will be hardest to hide. The blue-black dye should be painted with Dermacolour D32, Orange or Veil Rose with a small brush, before applying the matching skin shade. Red can be obliterated with Dermacolour 1742 or Veil Olive. Large tattoos are best covered with a natural or stipple sponge in the matching skin tone after the detailed brushwork has been completed.

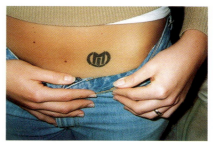

**Covering a tattoo
Before**

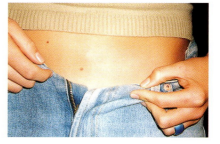

After

Covering an indented scar

1   First cover the scar with the shade which matches the surrounding skin tone.
2   Use a colour slightly paler than the matching skin shade and with a small brush apply a thin line around the inside edge of the scar. Tap it with your fingertip to blend and set in the usual way.
3   Using a slightly darker cream than the matching skin shade, apply a thin line around the outside of the scar. Blend it in by tapping lightly with your finger and set in the usual way.

Highlighting and shading after covering with the matching skin tone can often make a scar look less indented and the surrounding area look as if it protrudes less.

A protruding scar

The opposite method to covering an indented scar is required here.

1 Cover with the matching skin shade.
2 Using a shade of cream slightly darker than the matching skin tone, paint a line on the inside edge of the scar. Tap to blend with a fingertip and set in the usual way.
3 Use a lighter shade of cream and paint a line on the outside edge of the scar. Tap with fingertip to blend and set in the usual way.

Filling in a beardline

For a man who has bare patches of skin in his beardline, there is a greyish colour camouflage cream by Covermark which is made for this purpose. All the ranges do black and white, which can be mixed together with a little brown to get the authentic colour of a shaven beardline.

To apply the colour after matching it to the rest of the beardline, use a natural or stipple sponge. Test on the back of your hand and then stipple a tiny amount onto the patch, until the area blends in with the rest of the beardline. Finally, powder, brush off excess powder and use a dampened piece of cottonwool to thoroughly set the area.

Cross-infection

There is always the danger of cross-infection when using brushes and sponges for conveying make-up from the product to the skin. It is important that tools and products are kept scrupulously clean. Sponges and brushes should be washed in soap and water followed by a mild antiseptic solution before further use. Orange sticks and palette knives should be used for transferring the creams from their containers to a clean plate before mixing. It is the same for all make-up – but when you are covering a cold sore or any other skin blemish it is very important to be particularly careful. For this reason it is best to use cottonwool to powder the area, or a disposable powder puff, which can be thrown away after use.

Removal of camouflage creams

A simple bland cleansing cream, with no fragrance, is suitable for removing the camouflage creams. Damp cottonwool is good for wiping off the cream, followed by a mild toner such as rosewater with a little witch hazel or glycerine. Cotton buds can also be used for tiny areas and thrown in the wastebin after use.

The ability of a make-up artist to eliminate or tone down skin problems with the use of camouflage creams is definitely empowering in the workplace. In fashion work you can conceal a spot when normal cosmetic concealers fail to do the job, or cover shaving rashes on actors' faces without fear of infecting the area, which normal cosmetics might do. Camouflage skills are an extra tool for the make-up artist, even if they do not work in the world of clinics and hospitals.

For those who have an affinity with this type of work and choose to specialise in skin camouflage, the best way to begin is to attend a course and learn the basic skills. The various manufacturers of camouflage creams sometimes hold courses to demonstrate their products. The Association of Skin Camouflage, and the Red Cross can both supply helpful information. There are also courses for beauty therapists which include skin camouflage, and of course the clinics and burns units in city hospitals. What could be more rewarding than to earn a living by helping others to develop their confidence and rebuild their self-esteem in order to reintegrate into society?

Working in fashion and beauty

3

Introduction

The *fashion industry* is led by the media, designers, advertisers, manufacturers, stylists, models, make-up artists, hairdressers and photographers. They all feed off each other, taking their inspiration from street and pop culture, history, fine art and changes in society, to feed the public's demand for new trends. This is a competitive world – to be on top you need to be not just good but excellent.

The make-up artist works with highly creative people who are passionate about fashion. The models, photographers, stylists and make-up artists are all freelance, often with the same agencies, and tend to work together. To be successful the make-up artist needs to work the circuit, which is London, New York, Paris and Milan. This includes editorial work as well as the fashion shows. The fashion world is international, knowing no boundaries.

As a fashion make-up artist you must be recognised as 'sexy', 'minimalist', 'classic', 'edgy', 'funky', 'grunge', beauty, etc. The make-up artists are then catalogued and will have their own lines of work, making it easy for their agents to 'sell' them to big clients. In this way a make-up artist becomes 'bankable'. There is no age limit so long as you are up to date in the whole context of fashion. This means knowing who are the latest models, trends, designers, products, etc. The most successful clique of make-up artists creates the looks that provide inspiration in print and shows across the world, influencing a generation of fashion enthusiasts.

Tip

- Know your trade
- Be professional
- Clean presentation of self and make-up kit
- Sharp make-ups
- Pleasant and relaxed with everyone
- Up to date with make-up houses and cosmetic products

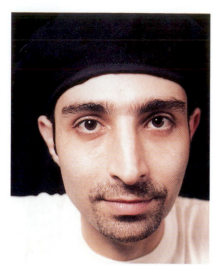

James Anda

Case Profile
James Anda, Make-up artist

How and when did you start in the business?
I enrolled for the Delamar Academy of Make-up where I was trained for three months. I started in 1990, I assisted Laurie Starrett for two years and then went out on my own.

Was there a turning point in your career?
After three years working and various tests for photographers, I did a beauty session for *Harper's Bazaar*, that changed my whole career.

What do you consider to be important qualities for a make-up artist?
Be clean in appearance and work, be fast and tidy, always be on time and know your trade by heart.

How has your career changed your life?
Working in fashion has allowed me to have a great lifestyle, which otherwise would be impossible to obtain and understand.

What have been your most satisfying jobs?
Working with people with whom I have worked for years, who have become like my family, my closest friends.

What advice would you give to young people entering the industry?
Follow your dream until it becomes a reality, never give up and most importantly really enjoy it.

Do you think the TV/film/theatre world is glamorous?
It is very glamorous and very real as well.

What would you consider to be the best and worst aspects of being a make-up artist?
Travelling and seeing all the best places for free is the best aspect and the worst is the food on location.

Kinds of fashion work

Fashion work is of several kinds, each with its own technical requirements:

- portrait (editorial) and advertising
- fashion shows
- music videos
- catalogue photography

Portrait (editorial) and advertising

This area of fashion includes all magazine art 'print work' and is high profile for the make-up artist, but not as well paid as the other areas. Most make-up artists compete for editorial because it enhances their reputation and they get a *tear sheet* for their book. It puts them in the public eye and can lead to other opportunities.

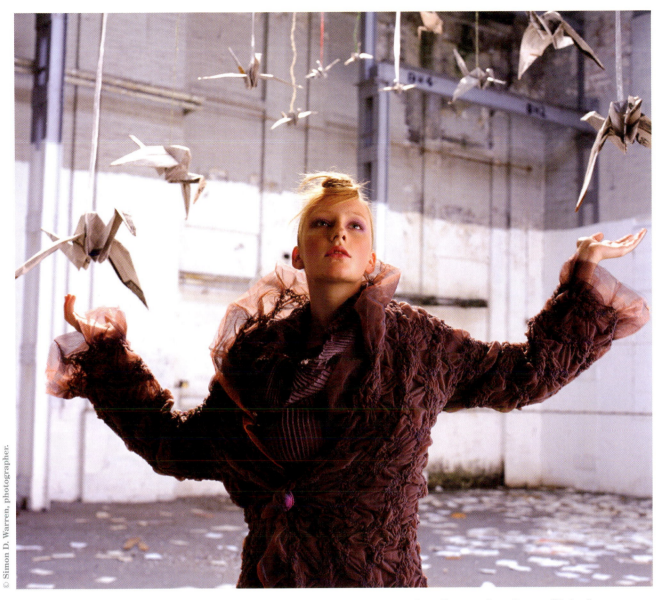

© Simon D. Warren, photographer.

Make-up artist Jo Frost using MAC for Spring/Summer 2002 Lezley George brochure. Hair James Rowe. Set design Alex Jeffrey. Styling Robin Easterby. Model Lucy Mayers at Take Two.

Some fashion make-up artists have become *personal make-up artists* on feature films through making up leading film actors on editorial jobs. The actor will request that person (through their agent) and the film company agrees if the actor has enough clout.

Other fashion make-up artists have created their own *make-up ranges* through contacts made during editorial work. The cosmetic companies compete for a credit in the magazine and are happy to give away free make-up in order to endorse their products, so the make-up artist usually has relationships with the most popular make-up lines.

The standard working day is 9.30am to 5.30pm and editorial work can be on location or in the studio. The make-up artist works with the stylist, photographer and models to create a look that is

Case Profile
Jo Frost, Make-up artist

How long have you been working in the industry?
Since the end of 1998.

How did you get into it?
My whole education history and working life was focused on fashion prior to becoming a professional make-up artist. I have always been obsessed with cosmetics and did projects and shows for a flatmate who was on a make-up course when I was a fashion student. Whilst working as a fashion buyer I began to buy cosmetics for the stores in addition to garments and began to mix with people in the industry. As my passion developed, it became apparent that I had to make a career change so I enrolled on a course with Penny.

What or who has been your most significant project?
There has been no one project that I would single out. I believe there is always more to achieve and a higher quality of work to pursue.

What do you enjoy most about your work?
I get a great buzz when I am working with a team that connects really well and has great energy. My most satisfying jobs have been those when the team vibe was really positive and I have built up relationships with those people. Editorial is my favourite work because you can push things much further to create incredible images. Whilst the photographs can be amazing this is not a glamorous business particularly for the models as all the clothes are shot one season ahead, so in the middle of summer you are shooting winter coats and in March you are shooting summer stock in a freezing location. I also enjoy the intimacy of the job – you work almost within kissing distance of your 'model' and communication with the rest of the team is paramount.

And least?
The days can be extremely long. I regularly work 12-hour days for fashion and pop promos are often longer.

What advice would you give to people trying to get into this area of work now?
This business is extremely competitive so never become complacent. Work is definitely affected by your contacts and will increase gradually as you meet more people and they get to know you. Initially you have to test all the time to get your book together and then get good editorial work before you can get an agent. Having an agent helps, but you must make sure that they understand the kind of work you want to do. Assisting is important after college, as it is a great way of continuing to learn, especially at London Fashion Week, which is incredibly inspiring.

Being a make-up artist is not just about doing make-up. You should emotionally boost the model/singer/actress and help prepare them for being in front of the camera – if they feel comfortable they look better. Face massages can help as they improve circulation in the skin and release stressed muscles – a relaxed model will give more to the camera and will naturally glow. You should always be aware of what is going on and anticipate things, just because you have finished the make-up do not assume that your day is over. Always be calm (even if you are having a stressed moment) and helpful by contributing to the team. Every day should be a good one, have fun and love what you do.

It is the best job in the world though as you meet interesting people and create beautiful pictures, it is challenging and exciting but can be stressful and tiring, but the buzz is the best thing in the world.

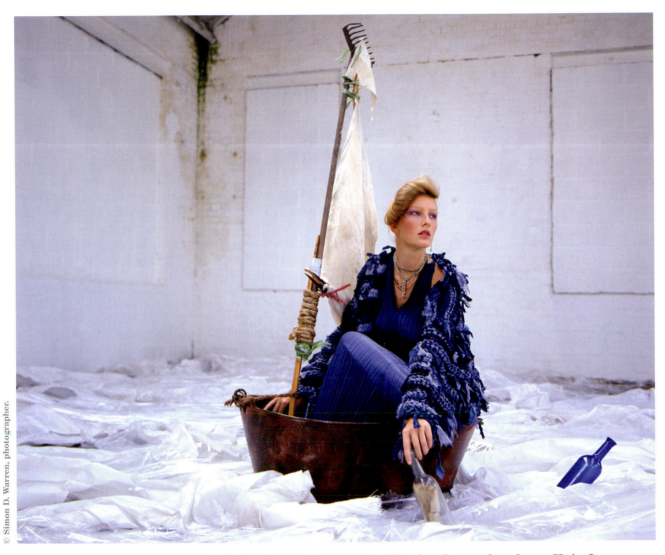

© Simon D. Warren, photographer.

Make-up artist Jo Frost using MAC for Spring/Summer 2002 Lezley George brochure. Hair James Rowe. Set design Alex Jeffrey. Styling Robin Easterby. Model Lucy Mayers at Take Two.

harmonious with the hair, clothes, models and lighting. This takes between one and three days, depending on the job. Typically, the make-up and hair would need to be done in one and a half hours with between one and three models. Because it is more competitive nowadays, the make-up artist is often responsible for the hair. The type of make-up could be artistic with no rules for the trendier magazines, or classic beauty, according to the client's brief.

Fashion shows

Known as *catwalk* or *runway*, this is where the trends are created by the designer and make-up artists. A complete fashion look is created to sell the clothes and every fashion show is covered extensively by the media. The shows are held three times a year, the main one being *couture* and the other two *prêt à porter* (ready to wear). They last for a week (seven days) and start in New York, followed by London, Paris and Milan. There are usually three shows a day at different venues.

Preparation and planning takes place three months before the show. The make-up artist has several meetings with the designer to understand the creative concept. Very often the designer and stylist will show the make-up artist various aids they have used to inspire them whilst working on the collection. They may be scraps of fabric, pictures, reference books, period or futuristic drawings – known as mood boards.

The make-up artist will then demonstrate the make-up ideas. When all has been agreed, the make-artist will show the rest of the make-up team what to do. There are usually four other make-up artists and hair stylists, plus three assistants. On the day of the show the team start to get the models ready at 4 am to be ready by 10 am. The same make-up team will often rush to the next two shows to work for other designers.

The make-up artists for top fashion designers often become well known in their own right through the exposure generated by the fashion editors who promote the shows in the media. Essential qualities for this type of work are:

- empathy with the designer's style
- being creative and coming up with new ideas
- fast and confident application of make-up

Trendy make-up

Trendy make-up is a fast-moving fashion style, meaning that it will last around three months. A magazine will use an idea for one issue and it may or may not catch on in the market. Usually this make-up will be so extreme that it will not suit the general public. Trendy make-up is designed to look at rather than to wear in everyday life.

There are no rules for this type of make-up as long as the shape suits the face. All kinds of materials may be used in different colours and textures. The normal rules of fashion make-up are deliberately broken to achieve a look that is artistic, ironic, humorous or challenging. Since anything goes, the make-up artist might use a combination of false eyelashes, sticking lipstick or paper on the eyelids and a combination of grease, powder and glitter. Even casualty effects and bald caps may be combined for an unusual effect. The idea is put into practice, seen in a magazine or on a runway, and then becomes history. As fashion takes ideas from the past, this creative industry moves in a fabulous circle – what goes around comes around.

Music videos

Music promos or music videos play an important role in promoting a new single or album, usually for TV broadcast. The band or individual artiste performs to their own soundtrack with dancers or crowd artists in a particular setting. The theme may be dreamt up by the record company or the musical performer. There is a director, a storyboard to show the action (not always) and the whole show is like a mini-film lasting for just minutes – the length of the soundtrack – according to the concept. It could involve animals, children or models; the music company hires in whatever or whoever is needed. The make-up/hair artist gets assistants to help and takes instructions from the director. Sometimes the make-up artist is from TV or film if the look is to be theatrical. Very often a fashion make-up artist is hired if the lead performer wants to update his image.

Music videos are fun to work on and often call for invention and versatility. Pop stars and musicians tend to start work at 4 pm and carry on all night for days at a time. To work in the music business, the make-up artist needs a sense of style, flexibility and stamina.

Catalogue photography

This area is probably the best paid of all fashion work but is not as prestigious as fashion or editorial. The shoots are usually in tropical locations where the light is beautiful. The make-up artist and models are booked for between ten and fifteen days. Locations tend to be somewhere hot with a beach or picturesque village. Normally there are one to three models to make up, with the look being changed to suit throughout the day. Work begins at 7 am to catch the light, with a break between 11 am and 3.30 pm when the light becomes too harsh. The make-up artist retouches the models' make-up and hair and they work again between 4 pm and 7.30 pm until the light has gone. Work continues in this way for 15 days. The type of make-up is always classic and very natural looking. This is the most minimal make-up in fashion. Many make-up artists like catalogue work because it is well paid and involves travelling to exotic places.

The agent

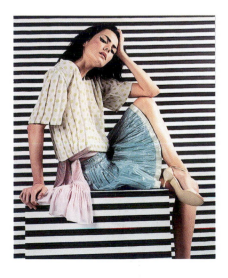

In order to be successful, all fashion make-up artists need an agency to represent them. Having an agent gives the artists credibility that they are reliable and know their trade. The agency promotes the make-up artists' careers putting out their name through its contacts and sending their portfolios to prospective clients. The top model agencies also represent make-up artists and hairdressers, so an editor or advertising company may book everyone for the job from the same agency. If a make-up artist gets to work well with a top model, their careers will progress together – on the fashion shows and doing editorial, TV and film work.

Fashion is a mixture of art and business. Since most make-up artists are creative people concentrating on their art, they need an agent for the business side of things. The agency negotiates rates of payment and organises meetings with photographers, editors and public relations companies, or exposure in beauty and fashion magazines. The *commission* taken by agents varies in different countries, for example, London agents take 20 per cent; Paris agents take 15 per cent; Milan agents take between 40 and 50 per cent.

Getting the right agent is a competitive area amongst make-up artists. The agencies want the best make-up artists. Everyone wants the best representation for themselves and it is never easy. To be taken on by an agent, it is essential to have a good *portfolio* of work to show what you can do. This means doing *test shots* with photographers for no fee in the hope of getting pictures for your book. In this way the make-up artist learns the trade. It is ironic, but an agent doesn't usually take someone on until they have built up a bit of a reputation and can bring their own contacts to the agency. However, many agents complain that they spend several years building up a make-up artist's career, making them *bankable*, only to see the person poached by a rival agency. When you are successful everyone wants you.

Professionalism

Presentation is always important for the make-up artist, but for the artist working in fashion it is crucial. You must always look presentable and your equipment must be scrupulously clean.

Planning too is vital. Be sure to prepare thoroughly in advance. Make written notes of what you will need and assemble all the necessary materials before the shoot. In planning the make-up, remember to think about light and shade, even when using colour.

Tip

When maintaining the make-up for a shoot, always apply more powder to the model before it looks necessary. This way the make-up does not have time to deteriorate.

Activity – Planning light and shade

Look at a colour palette. Think of it as shade and highlight. If you were to take a photograph of it using black-and-white film, which colours should show as shadows, which as mid-tones and which as highlights? Which tones are lighter and which darker than the foundation colour you are working with?

Preparing the make-up

Always try to make life easy for yourself – don't complicate things unnecessarily. As far as possible, plan everything in advance: the shape of the eye colour, the type of make-up, the colours, base and liner you will use, and so on. You should know before you start exactly what the end result will be. For all make-up, the basic questions to ask yourself are these:

1 Why am I using this product?
2 Why am I applying it to this area?
3 Why have I chosen this colour?
4 What will the result look like?

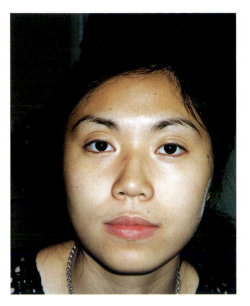

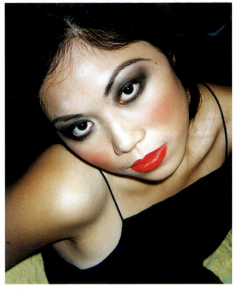

Before

After
Make-up by Kulwadee Songsiri.
Model: Sally Studley

Applying the make-up

Tip

If the model has dry skin, use a cream foundation: panstik is suitable for dry skin. If the model has greasy skin, use a water-based liquid foundation.

When testing the foundation to find the right colour, apply a little on the model's forehead or jawline.

The foundation

Choosing the foundation

In photographic work it is common to select a foundation one shade darker than the natural skin tone. If the shot involves exposed body areas, always be guided by the skin tone on the neck, chest, arms and legs.

'White' skins tend to have more yellow in them than one might imagine. Often they are darker in the centre of the face and lighter around the edges.

'Black' skins tend to have more orange in them than one might suppose. They are often lighter in the centre of the face and darker around the edges.

In choosing the foundation, the object is to select an in-between shade, one that will balance the skin tone to achieve an even base. On the whole it is usually better to choose a slightly darker base for white skins and a slightly lighter one for black skins.

Blending the foundation

Blend the foundation well around the edges of the face and on the neck area. Don't apply much foundation to the cheeks and make sure that what you do apply fades down the sides of the face until the edge disappears.

Apply foundation right into the eyebrows to avoid edges appearing. The brows can be coloured in afterwards.

If any imperfections show, apply more foundation. If you have worked the foundation in well – a little at a time, concentrating on one area before beginning the next – it should be right first time. Always work to the same routine: *forehead, centre, sides, neck*.

Powdering

To set the foundation and prevent shine, use a little powder, but not too much at a time. The foundation must not 'clog'. The powder blots any superfluous moisture. Be careful not to put too much powder on the eye areas.

Eyeshadows

Brush the eyelids to remove creases before applying eyeshadow. *Press* the colour on exactly where you want it. *Do not flick the brush*. Blend the edges with a clean brush to diffuse the lines.

The lips

To paint the lips, face the model straight on. When using a strong colour such as red, use a *lip pencil* to get a perfect shape before applying the lipstick. For a natural effect, use a soft coral pink and add some powder: mix these on a palette to give a soft matt appearance.

Always use the same *lip brush*, which should be shaped, to apply a lipstick. Using a favourite brush in this way will give you maximum control. When applying lipstick, start at the corner of the mouth. *Roll* the brush, following the shape of the lips.

Lip pencils

Sometimes matt-looking lips are in fashion, sometimes glossy. When using gloss, the lips need a firm borderline to prevent the gloss from sliding. Strong-coloured lipstick glosses need a matching lip pencil outline applied first.

If using pale or natural-coloured gloss, use a brown pencil to outline the lips first: this adds definition.

For actresses of mature years whose lipstick would otherwise 'bleed' into fine lines around the mouth, lip pencil can be used to outline the lips.

Lip sealers

Lip sealers are products made to coat the lipstick with a transparent liquid which seals the lip colour and prevents it from smudging. They tend to sting the lips when first applied, but are useful in scenes or shots where the actress has to eat, drink or kiss as they help to prevent the lipstick from moving.

The skin

Blusher

Blusher should be placed depending on whether the make-up is for colour photography or black and white.

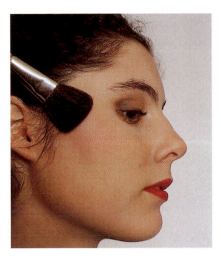

Applying blusher for colour photography

- **Colour photography** Apply blusher along the cheekbones to highlight the shade of the overall skin tone.
- **Black-and-white photography** Apply blusher beneath the cheek bones to shape them.

As the blusher is being used to create shading, the *shade* of the blusher is more important than its colour. Often a pinky rust colour is useful, blended well so that it is not too strong.

The use of blushers

Blusher, or cheek colour, used to be known as *rouge* or *carmine*. It was obtained by crushing cochineal (a Mexican insect) into a red powder. Nowadays there is a vast selection of powders and creams, in every shade and tone. Sometimes it is difficult to choose which type to use.

- **Powder blushers** These are easy to apply and can be added at the end of the make-up for added warmth and colour.
- **Cream blushers** These need to be blended with a sable brush and tend to survive longer than powder types. Cream rouge is better on dry skin or on cheeks that are blemished, as it is easier to blend. Cream is also more waterproof.
- **Powder/cream blushers** This type of blusher is applied like a cream, but dries to a matt finish like powder.

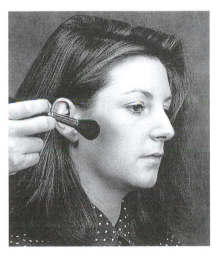

Applying blusher for black-and-white photography

Choosing the blusher

The choice of blusher depends on the colour of the skin tone:

- **Black skin tones** These need brown shades, so choose orange-browns and red-browns to enhance the skin colour. Avoid bright pinks, as these look unnatural.
- **Dark olive skin tones** These look best with brownish blushers, shades of terracotta and russet pinks.
- **Pink skin tones** These may not need blusher at all, if the cheeks are already pink or if they tend to blush easily. Peach tones can be used to play down the colour if it is too rosy.
- **Golden skin tones** These look good with coral and peach colours on the cheeks. It is good to use pinks to offset the skin tone if this is on the sallow side.
- **Ivory and pale skins** These should not have strong cheek colours added. Shades of beige pinks and pale pinks harmonise well with this type of skin tone, which is delicate and often appears translucent.

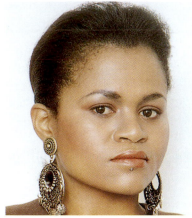

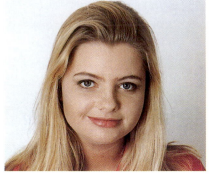

A pink skin tone

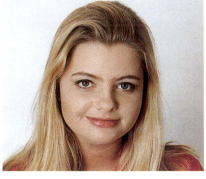

A black skin tone

An ivory skin tone

Effects of photographic lighting on make-up

Make-up artists work with photographers, who generally have preferred styles of working. It is up to the make-up artist to adapt to the way the photographer uses lights. In general, the stronger the light, the more it bleaches out the make-up.

The lights in photography draw attention to any shine, so you must always use matt colours with no glitter or shine in the pigment. The photographer will decide where he wants a shiny effect, if at all. Always stay close to the camera in case you are needed to retouch the make-up.

A fashion make-up

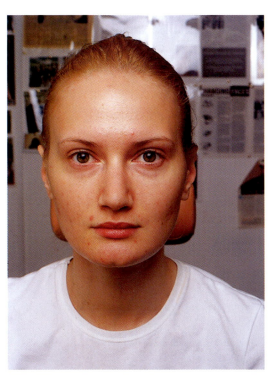

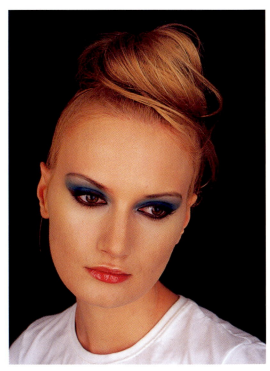

Before

After

Make-up for advertising

Basic principles apply here as elsewhere. Here are a few additional points:

- **Housewives** Basic 'housewife' make-up must not overpower the product being advertised.

- **Men** When making up men, remember that the make-up must be invisible. Cover spots and blemishes and keep make-up to a minimum.

- **Children** Children may need rosier cheeks, For a natural look, use grease rather than powder blushers.

Your own professional image

Tip

Always carry some business cards with your telephone number and address to hand out when requested.

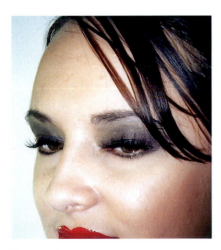

Eye make-up

In fashion and advertising, the way you look is more important than any other area of the media. Your choice of hairstyle, make-up, clothes and the products you carry in your make-up box will all be seen as examples. The following hints may be useful:

1 Keep abreast of fashion and try to be aware of coming fashions. Everyone working in fashion is fashion conscious – don't fall behind.

2 Try out new products continually. Don't be afraid of rapid changes in fashion.

3 Keep updating your skills on refresher courses.

4 Build up good relationships with the models and photographers you work with. If you are courteous and professional, they will notice.

5 How you look, how you present yourself, how you act, how you move and how you speak will all make an impression on those you work for and with. The impression you wish to convey is of being competent, friendly and trustworthy.

Alternative styles in eye make-up

Fashions constantly change, so it is impossible to define or pin down a particular effect as being the current fashion. Fashion always borrows from the past and there are definite influences from other decades, adapted and changed to suit the mood of the present. The following activities allow you to practice alternative styles in eye make-up.

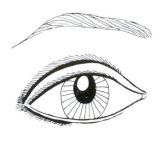

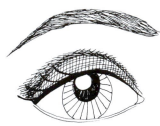

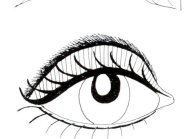

Alternative styles in eye make-up

Activity – 1980s eye make-up (natural)

1 Draw a dark colour in the socket line using a matt, compressed powder eyeshadow.
2 Use the same product as an eyeliner, drawing it across the lid above the eyelashes and underneath the eyes at the outer corners.
3 Blend these lines up to meet the socket line and blend them away and outwards – but no further than the point indicated by the nose-to-eye measuring technique.

Activity – 1990s eye make-up (strong)

1 Mix a dark brown or grey compressed powder eyeshadow with water.
2 Apply it all over the eyelids, blending the edges.
3 If you find the eyeshadow difficult to blend (damp eyeshadow dries quickly), try pressing the powder with your brush, rather than stroking it on. Press the eyeshadow powder up and over the socket lines.
4 Apply eyeliner, blending well.

Activity – A 1960s look

1 Apply white eyeshadow to the eyelids.
2 Draw in the socket lines using black pencil.
3 Blend the socket lines gently.
4 Apply grey eyeshadow to the eyelids.
5 Add white eyeshadow to the eyebrow bones.
6 Attach false eyelashes.
7 Apply eyeliner.

Fashion make-up

It is easier to illustrate beauty than high fashion in a textbook because the first is classic and the second is here today and gone tomorrow. Fashion trends are meant for weekly or monthly magazines – not books that take a year to produce. The same applies to films, which is why you don't see many trendy fashion make-ups on the cinema screen. A film set in a distant period is often responsible for setting a fashion trend, never the other way round.

The fashion make-ups shown here are the current trends in London and Paris, January 2002. By the time you see these pictures they may have become historical make-ups. The original early 1990s make-ups have come round again in fashion revival style. So who knows? That is the whole point of the fickle and fascinating face of fashion.

Fashion make-ups by James Anda

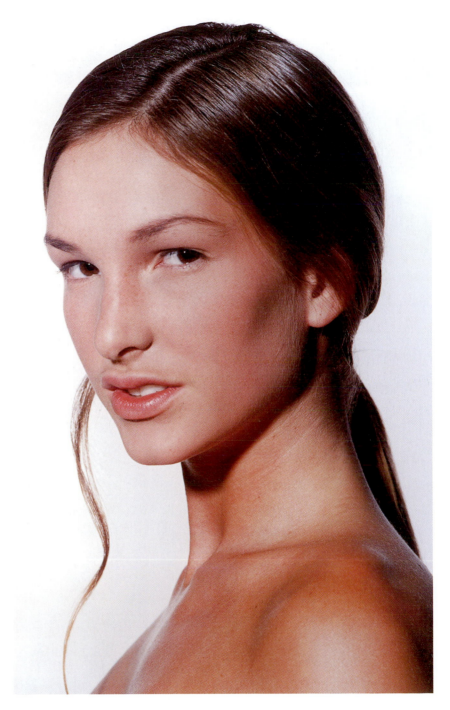

Beauty: Classic style on a 17-year-old model

1 Translucent powder was applied all over the face.
2 Brown powder used to define the eyebrows.
3 A peach-coloured blusher was brushed across the cheeks with a soft brush.
4 Lip gloss was applied to the lips for a natural looking shine.

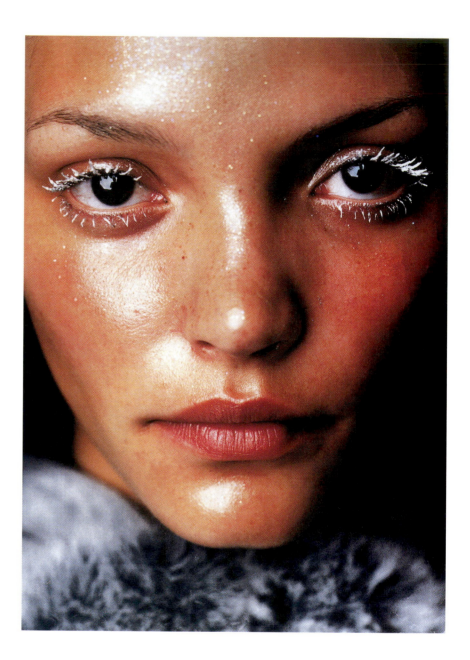

Fashion show make-up

1 James used coconut oil all over the face, applied very lightly with a sponge.

2 Black mascara was used on the top and bottom eyelashes.

3 Once the mascara was dry, a white water colour (as used in body painting) was applied on top of the lashes.

4 Glitter dust was used all over the face. To do this, the glitter is held in the palm of the hand and blown towards the face. The model should close her eyes whilst this is happening. The glitter will stick to the coconut oil.

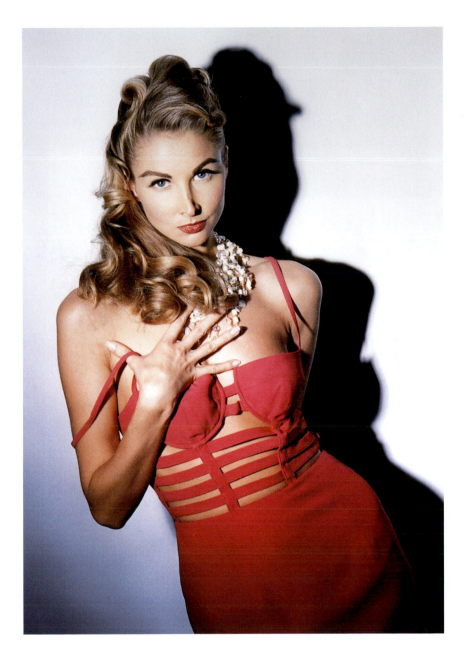

Traditional 1950s make-up with modern hair

1 An ivory liquid foundation was applied all over the face with a sponge.
2 Translucent powder was used to set the foundation for a matt finish using a powder puff.
3 Brown powder was applied to the eyebrows to define the shapes.
4 Black eyeliner was applied close to the lashes for a 1950s look.
5 False eyelashes were fitted and applied to add to the film star look.
6 Peach blusher was brushed across the cheeks.
7 The lips were painted with red lipstick to complete the look.
8 The hair was set on heated rollers in a modern shape, keeping the feel of a 1950s movie star but in a modern way.

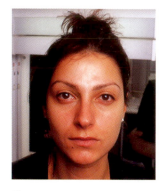

Step 1

Make-up suitable for beauty, wedding and catalogue work

1 Model without make-up.

2 Foundation applied using light olive ultra fluid foundation.

3 It was not necessary to use concealer under the eyes as the model's skin colour is good.

4 Yellow translucent powder was used to set the foundation and match the skin tone.

5 Use black or brown powder to shape the eyebrows.

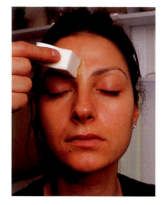

Step 2

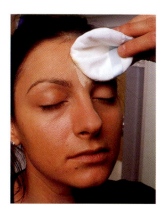

Step 3

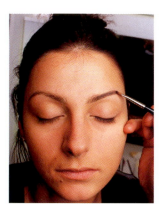

Step 4

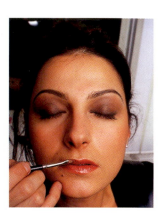

Step 5

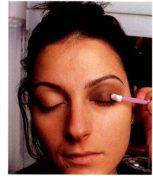

Step 6

6 The eyelids are brushed with brown powder and blended well to give a perfect natural look.

7 Black powder was used to draw the eye lines and blended well.

8 Black mascara was applied to the top lashes only.

9 Terracotta and a natural shade of blusher were mixed and used on the cheeks.

10 Lips with shine only to 'lift' the make up.

The hair is pulled back for a clean sharp look and an elegant finish. Water spray and gel were used for achieving this classic look.

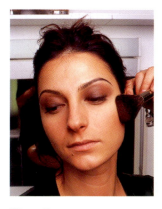

Step 7

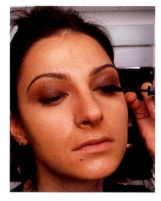

Step 8

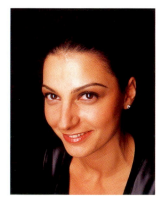

Step 9

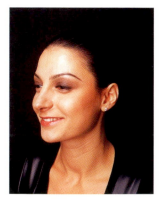

Step 10

Smokey eyes

The smokey-eyed look has been used for more than 30 years in the fashion industry and is still used commercially today – just updating the colour of blush and lips to give a more modern version.

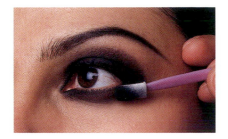

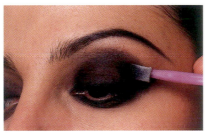

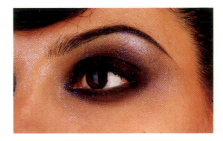

1 Foundation applied using light olive ultra fluid foundation. Again, concealer was not necessary.

2 Translucent powder matching skin tone is used to set the foundation.

3 Eyebrows are darkened more than usual with black powder or pencil to balance the heavy eyeshadow.

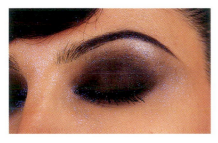

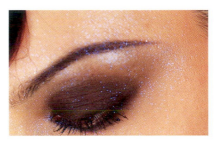

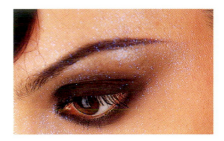

4 The whole eye area is darkened with black eyeshadow in a round shape and blended.

5 Black mascara on top and bottom eyelashes.

6 Very pale blush.

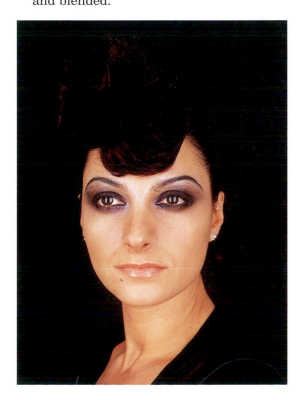

7 Shine on lips to balance the whole make up and avoid a theatrical look.

The hair is inspired by the Punk movement, but more 'relaxed', to suit the extreme black eyes, plus glitter dust on top as a final finish. Backcombing and use of hair lacquer to bring the hair forward to give a dramatic Punk modern look.

Model Hale

Make-up for commercials

The companies that produce television commercials often hire the same crews to ensure a high level of expertise. The make-up artists can be from any of the different areas of work – fashion, theatre, television or film – depending on the required look. The budgets are usually generous and the scale of the production, particularly for a rich client, is often similar to an epic mini-film.

Many film directors started their working lives in commercials, for example, Ridley Scott, Alan Parker, David Putnam and Hugh Hudson. It has often been said that the high standards of commercials in Britain provide an excellent training ground for future work in cinematography.

Commercial for Carling
© Michael Lewin

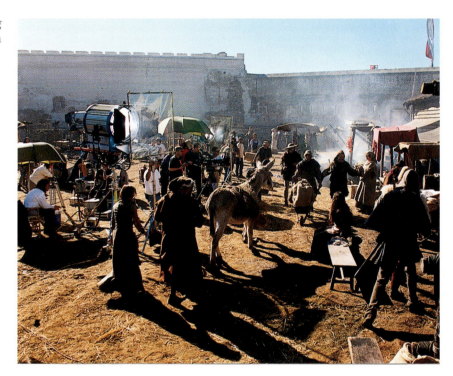

The end product in *commercial advertising* may be for television or the cinema. Either way, it is vital to bear in mind that each and every detail counts. Realism is not what is sought. If someone hits his head, for example, no bruise will be required. No one will show any blemishes. Children will look natural and perfect. The actors for such productions are cast very carefully – often they are models, chosen for their looks. Nevertheless, corrective make-up will sometimes be needed.

Working in a team

Filming commercials is extremely expensive, so everyone involved must work swiftly and confidently. Often the clients are present,

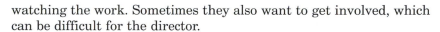

watching the work. Sometimes they also want to get involved, which can be difficult for the director.

As the make-up artist, you will need to be relaxed and friendly with a lot of people, many of whom may be total strangers. In contrast to film, television and theatre work, the cast and crew for a commercial are thrown together simply for one day and must 'gel' immediately. Commercial production companies like to use the same people repeatedly to reduce this problem.

No one in this sort of work can afford to have an 'off' day: others depend on you. You need to cultivate a professional attitude and a willingness to attempt anything as asked. Usually there won't even be a rehearsal. *Children and animals* often form part of the cast of commercials. To be able to entertain them between takes is a real asset in a make-up artist.

Planning

You should be ready to create any effect required. You may find yourself providing fashion make-up for a beautiful model in a yoghurt advertisement one day and wigs and facial hair for a period piece the next.

Usually you will be able to find a plan for the commercial in the form of a *storyboard*, a scene-by-scene drawing showing the sequence of shots and what will appear in each.

On the set

Unless there are a great many actors, which would be unusual, one make-up artist will be expected to do the make-up and hair for the whole cast. Hands are especially important in commercials; most actors will need a *manicure*. There may be a 'hand artist' for certain shots, but this is uncommon. You should always be prepared, with a manicure set, nail-varnish remover and several shades of varnish in your kit box. If one of the cast is playing a mother, she will probably need colourless nail varnish.

Never use a foundation on young children. If the director says a child's face is too pale, resist applying a tan base immediately. Instead try putting warmth into the skin by stippling the cheeks and forehead with a little blusher or warm brown. Bear in mind too that a young child will quickly get quite warm under the lights. Wait to see whether this happens before rushing in with make-up. Work with the lighting cameraman, who is usually able to be very helpful in achieving the desired effect. Don't overlook body make-up and never forget the hands and ears. Remember – with commercials, it's all in the detail.

Tip

When working with young children, some crayons and paper will help to keep them from getting bored.

Tip

Sometimes an actor may nick himself when shaving. A medical 'new skin' is available from chemists and is useful to have in your kit box.

It is useful to carry aspirins or paracetamol in your kit box in case an artiste has a headache.

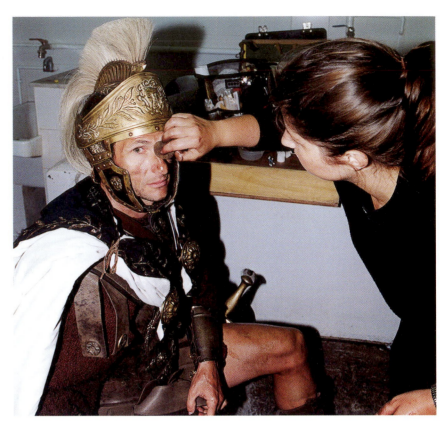

Make-up artist Rebecca Burge working on commercial for Swiss Milk 'Gladiator'

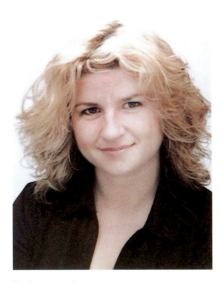

Rebecca Burge

Case Profile
Rebecca Burge, Make-up artist

How long have you been in the industry?
I have been a make-up artist in the Film Industry for about 5 years.

How did you get into it?
Whilst working as a location caterer on the television series *Sharpe*, the make-up designer, Julianne Chapman, told me I should become a make-up artist because I had the right qualities and temperament. She recommended me to the Make-up Centre and the rest is history.

What or who has been your most significant projects?
Make-up designer Patti Merchant and I were nominated for 'The best make-up and prosthetics' at the 1999 British Advertising Crafts Awards.

What do you enjoy most about your work?
I enjoy every aspect of my work. I don't even mind the getting up in the early morning! I love learning new skills and being challenged. I take great delight in doing intricate make-up's on individuals and take great pride in doing large, particularly period crowd scenes.

What advice would you give to people trying to get into this area of work now?
Don't give up if it is your dream, because every job is an achievement and a reward.

Body and face painting

4

Introduction

The art of body painting covers a vast area of painted effects and some make-up artists choose to specialise in this subject, working through an agent, usually in fashion and advertising. There are also many gifted make-up artists who include body painting as an additional skill that normally work in film and television. Body painting is the art of painting any effect from a simple tattoo on the arm to reproduction of a famous painting across an entire body or painting a model to look fully clothed. To be successful in this highly creative niche an arts background is needed, or at least a familiarity with the skills of drawing and painting.

Body painting

Since the process is very time consuming it is essential to plan the design on paper and then try it out on a mannequin or model before the shoot. This way problems can be overcome in advance.

The materials used for painting are special watercolours for the skin, available from professional make-up shops. These are supplied in liquids, creams and palettes of varied colours. The tools used to apply the body paints are various sponges, brushes, or any type of tool which gives the desired coverage, including airbrushing. Stencils are useful for repeat patterns; masking tape is good for a clean edge effect; natural or stipple sponges for **stippling** textures; and feathers may be used for marbling effects. For a statue effect it is best to use a large, bath-sized natural sponge to stipple the appearance of stone. **Chinese brushes** will also give a marble effect similar to using feathers. Specialist books on creating paint effects for furniture are useful. So long as you use watercolour make-up instead of paint, you can employ the same techniques for gilding, tortoise shell effects, etc.

For painting clothes on the body, an idea used frequently in photography and advertising, it is best to use sable artist's brushes, sponges and airbrushing techniques. In fact body painting is truly an art, giving enormous potential for freedom of expression and imaginative use of different make-up techniques.

Clown make-up

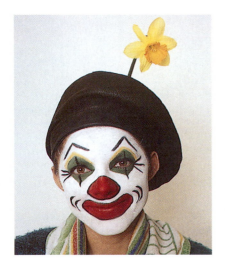

Clown make-up

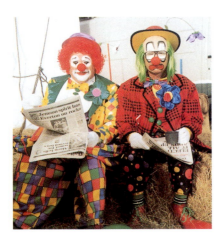

Clown make-up: Sid Little and Eddie Large as clowns

As well as being fun to do, clown make-ups are very good for practising balance and precision. The well-known types are the tramp and the whitefaced clown, but there is no such thing as a standard clown – each face should be individual to the performer.

The *tramp clown* doesn't have a white face. He is generally unshaven looking, with old, baggy clothes and a battered bowler hat. The eyebrows, eyes and mouth are painted and he has a bright red, bulbous nose. This can be made from half a table-tennis ball, stuck on the nose with **spirit gum**; or by slush-moulding for a rubber nose. The mouth is painted red or white and drawn very large, either turning up to look happy or down to look sad.

The *whitefaced clown* is more colourful, with primary colours being used to create the design. The outlines should be drawn in black pencil, with emphasis on the eyebrows, nose, eyes and mouth.

Planning the make-up

Clowns can be funny, sad, suspicious, elegant or tragic. Bald caps with crepe hair laid on in bright colours are useful to complete the look. White stocking-tops, pulled over the head to hide the hair, make good skullcaps. Eye markings are individual, but the black cross over the eyelids is well known, as are the painted teardrop and the raised eyebrows.

Before starting the make-up, draw the proposed clown design on paper, filling it in with coloured pencils to illustrate the final effect.

Applying the make-up

Draw the design on your model with an eyebrow pencil. If using a white base, choose a pancake: this is easy to wash off with soap and water. When the foundation is dry, finish with white talcum powder.

Pierrot and Pierrette

Pierrot has a plain white face. If the eyebrows of the man to be made up are too heavy, they should be eliminated by soaping them down and applying wax or eyebrow plastic on top. Using a clown's white pancake, paint the entire face with a damp sponge, and powder when dry with white or transparent powder. The eyebrows

Pierrot

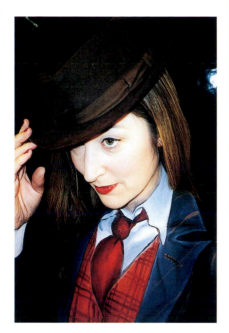

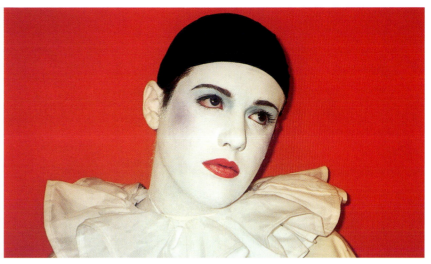

Painted clothes
Make-up artist Gemma
Richards. Model Poppy Hill

should be well arched and black. The lips should be painted bright red in Cupid's bow fashion. Add definition to the eyes with black pencil and two beauty spots to complete the look – one on the cheekbone near the eye, the other on the opposite side of the face, nearer the corner of the mouth. The man should wear a black skullcap, covering the hair.

For the Pierrette, the lady is made up to look as pretty as possible. Often she wears a hat.

Body art

Peacock

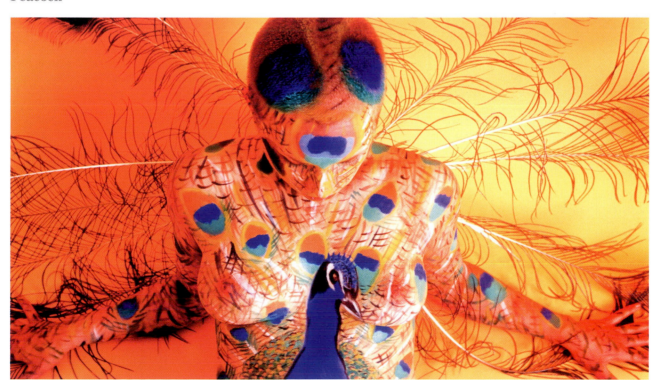

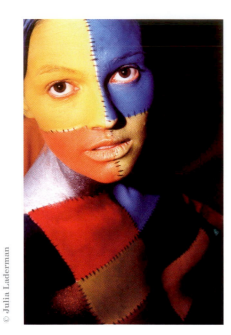

© Julia Laderman

Patchwork

Case Profile
Julia Laderman, Make-up artist

How and when did you start in the business?
I have been a practising make-up artist for over two years.

Was there a turning point in your career?
I would say it was launching myself into body art. I found that putting my energy into this was more rewarding for me than make-up. In particular, body painting pregnant women appeals to me the most.

What do you consider to be important qualities for a make-up artist?
Be friendly, personable and confident. You should also be flexible, patient and calm.

How has your career changed your life?
My life has become more exciting because my job has allowed me to work with a variety of people in places I would not have normally seen.

What have been your most satisfying jobs?
My most satisfying job was my very first one – I started as an assistant on a feature film and ended up as head of department. The original head had to leave, in extenuating circumstances, and I was fortunate to be in the right place at the right time.

What advice would you give to young people entering the industry?
Be patient and never give up, there is always something just around the corner.

Do you think the TV/film/theatre world is glamorous?
The film world is definitely not glamorous. In fact very few parts of being a make-up artist are glamorous. The two just don't go together.

What would you consider to be the best and worst aspects of being a make-up artist?
The best part of being a make-up artist is that each job brings new challenges and you are constantly learning. No two jobs are the same and there are many different fields in which one can specialise. The worst part is that you never know when that next job is! There is a lot of networking to be done and jobs tend to come from who you know and not what you know. It's not much fun carrying a heavy kit around either, so be warned!

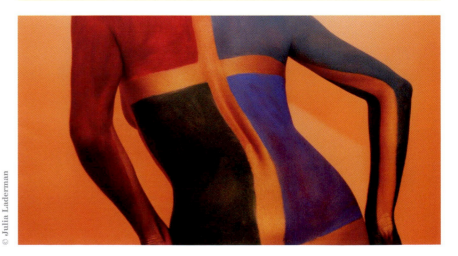

© Julia Laderman

Step-by-steps

Seahorse

1 I often find inspiration from nature. A seahorse fits perfectly down the centre of the spine.

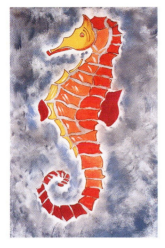 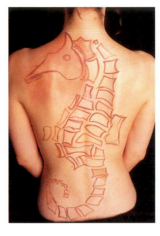 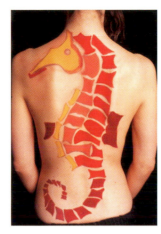 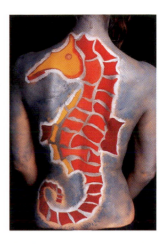

2 I first painted the seahorse on paper as a reference, using the colours that I had in mind.

3 I painted the outline of the seahorse onto the back with a fine brush and a pale aquacolour.

4 I then introduced reds, oranges and yellows using fine and wide angled brushes.

5 For the background, I use a soft small sponge and stippled blue, green and silver together. I outlined the seahorse with white and silver using a thin brush and blended with a larger brush.

6 Finally, using a wide paintbrush and **aquacolour**, I painted the hair and brought out the eye with blue pearls attached with double-sided sticky tape.

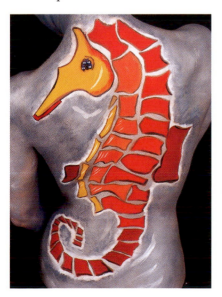 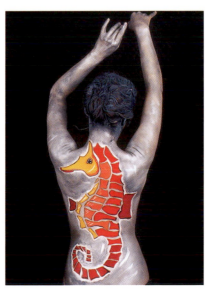 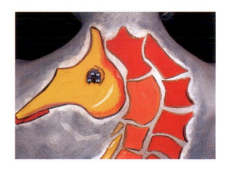

Make-up artist Julia Laderman
Model Avril Solomon

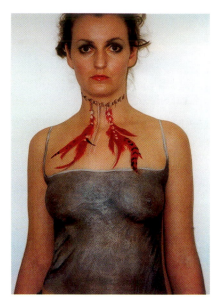

Make-up artist Francesca
Hingston

Lady with Feather Necklace

1   For this piece of work, I did the foundation colour on the torso using a natural sponge – for easy and less time consuming coverage, whilst still keeping to the feel of the material.

2   I used a mid-grey – so as to create a good base to paint on the highlights and shadows in detail.

3   For the folds in the material, I used a brush, blending the light into the shadow as smoothly as possible. The material I was aiming to recreate was very light and thin – I needed to transfer these delicate qualities into my work.

4   After I had done the detail, I carefully went over one more time with the sponge and completed the effect by stippling and filling in any gaps of colour.

5   The necklace was to be the main visual focus of the finished photograph. I used a medium-sized brush to paint the main shapes and colours, then continued to finish the piece with a very fine brush in order to create a realistic feather effect and add detail.

6   To finish, I applied talcum powder onto the paint.

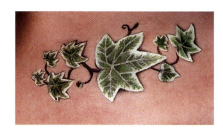

Make-up artist Francesca
Hingston

Ivy Detail on Back

1   I painted this piece from a real branch of ivy, to get the colours and shapes as true to life as possible. I wanted the finished photograph to give the optical illusion that a real branch of ivy was resting on the model's back – rather than being painted on.

2   In this project I used the lightest colour that was visible in the pattern of the ivy, to make my initial skeleton for the piece.

3   Then it was simply a matter of building up the colours how they naturally occurred on the plant. This was a good method to avoid the colours 'bleeding' into one another and losing their sharpness.

4   To finish off the piece, I applied a matching toned aquacolor to the model's skin, and used a sponge to go over the skin surrounding the painted design.

5   I used talcum powder over the paint to finish. This evens out the skin tone on camera and allows the focus to be on the design, rather than the surrounding skin.

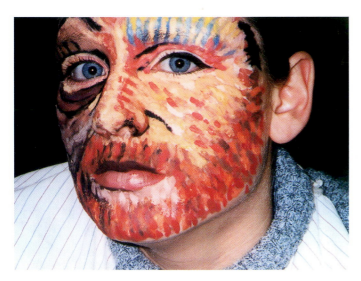

Make-up artist Francesca Hingston

Van Gogh Face Painting

1   The method I used to make the bodypaint (watercolour) seem more 3D and oil-paint like was to mix the paint with talcum powder.

2   I used a heavily laden, medium-sized brush to give the 'crusty' look on the overall effect.

3   I also tried to keep as much to van Gogh's style and use of colour as possible – making sure that I used slightly brighter and more vivid colours than one would think to use, so the colours were done justice in the finished photograph.

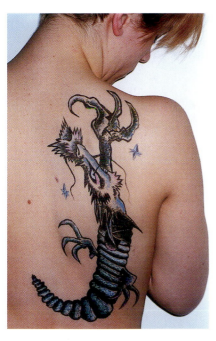

Make-up artist Francesca Hingston

Dragon Tattoo on Back

1   This design was inspired by a bodypainting from an advert I saw – I loved the composition of it and the use of black against pastel colours. So when I did this project I exaggerated the use of these two types of colours and added my own ideas to the design (extra detail, etc.).

2   This piece was all painted using a medium-sized brush for the majority and a fine brush for intricate detail.

3   Unlike my method for the ivy design, I started painting the design as I went along, rather than blocking it all before painting on the detail. This allowed me more scope to change things and to let the ideas that came into my mind be painted as they occurred. I feel this gave the finished piece more of a feeling of spontaneity rather than if I had planned it as much as the previous projects. It was an interesting style to develop, I thought.

4   To finish the piece and make it ready to be photographed, I did the same thing as with the ivy design. I used a matching aquacolor to even out the skin tone.

5   I used talcum powder and a puff to powder the whole design.

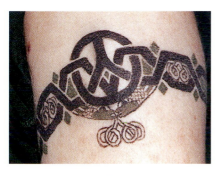

Make-up artist Francesca Hingston

Celtic Tattoo

1   This design was originally inspired by a ring I owned. The style is called a Celtic Knot and I thought that it would be a challenging project to do.

2   As the knot design itself was quite intricate, a fine brush was used to create it.

3   I mapped out the main part of the tattoo and then, once completed successfully, added my own ideas, which I had previously sketched down.

4   Like the Dragon tattoo, I wanted to add a bit more dimension to the design and increased use of colour – rather than having the whole tattoo black. This would also enhance it photographically.

5   To finish, I powdered it, but used no aquacolor. I wanted this project to look as if it could be a genuine tattoo. Therefore I didn't want the surrounding skin to look too 'flawless'.

Yin and Yang tattoo

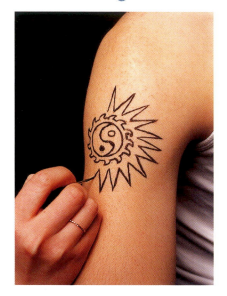

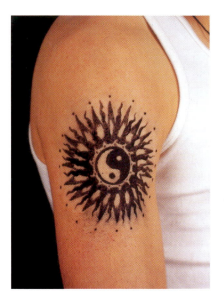

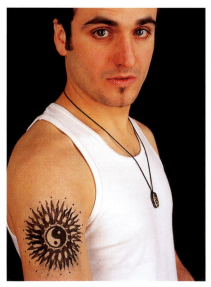

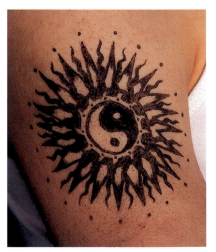

Make-up artist Francesca Hingston

This body art design is based on a yin yang symbol which represents balance and appeals to me because of the accuracy needed to reproduce it. The sun rays and other details add a tribal feel to it.

Since I was not working to a sketch design it was essential to have an accurate outline at the start. This was directly applied with a brush and black body paint. More black body paint is used to fill in the crux of the design. Details such as the sun rays have been added with a fine brush. The design is then powdered thoroughly to set it and make it look more like a tattoo.

Rough outline of owl project and comments

Budget

- I set out my own budget. (Always work to the budget set. If you know you are about to run over, discuss this with your make-up designer or producer.)
- Do the initial research and spend wisely. There is always an alternative so never purchase the first thing you see – shop around.
- Calculate each item and work within the budget. You will make your boss happier if you save money.
- This project was an owl – so obviously the one important item on the shopping list was the feathers.
- Try out the idea first if you can and purchase only a few items to start. Practise gluing some feather onto latex to start with.
- Find out if the piece has to be worn more than once. Consider other ways of making the piece within the budget.
- The project cost around £6.00.

Theme

- Choose your theme and work within the time allotted. If you have limited time, don't leave anything until the last minute as there are always hitches. I chose an owl for my piece and this was a challenge.
- If you can try out the materials on a trial/prep run, this makes the job easier – prepare and think in advance. Skin allergies, contact lenses, hot lights and costume changes can all be determining factors.

Make-up artist Shirley Brody

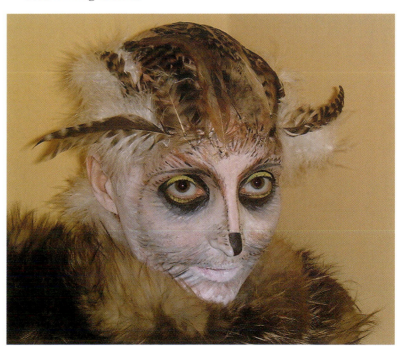

- This project took a day of preparations and a morning to apply.
- In a live situation (for theatre) where the actor performed several times in a row, twice a day, I would have to create much more of a hard-wearing piece.

Model

- When choosing the theme always consider the model/actor and tailor the theme around the face/body.
- My chosen model was very owl like in features with beautiful eyes and a fine shaped face so I had a good base to work with. In the real world you have no choices but the face you are given, so try and bring forward the features you want to strengthen and play down what is not so desirable.

Bald cap

- Make sure you have all the components ready and set out in an orderly fashion before your start.
- The bald cap was difficult in this case since my model had long, thick, black hair. She also had a low forehead, which meant unless I measured her head correctly the cap would be too small, which was exactly what happened. I had a big task in making it fit. All the feathers were stuck down individually and some were placed below the edge of the cap towards the bridge of her nose. I used watercolours, pan stick and powdered between layers to set each layer. I made sure the glue (spirit gum) was tacky prior to placing the feathers in position. I used a pair of tweezers to pick up the feathers and applied glue with a small stick to the spine of the feather for the first layer, and also applied a little glue to the bald cap. This made a solid base for what followed. I had to be very quick with the rest of the feathers and only applied the smallest amount of glue to them as I laminated a careful shape. After covering most of the head with feathers, I then applied a strip of feather down (purchased on the roll) to give a fluffy soft appearance. This also helped cover patches and reinforce it. I added large feathers each side of the forehead to imitate ears.

Make-up

As I mention above I used watercolours and panstik. I painted the entire face with small, fine, feather-like strokes to create a furry effect. I used her own eyebrows (thin brows did not need to be soaped out) for the heart shape and took this line round the inside of her face, using the chin for the point of the heart. Note that the beak is in the same plane as the brow. I did not use any moisturiser or toner prior to applying the make-up. The model's face was a perfect texture for applying the paint. I wanted a matt appearance – too oily a surface would have created the wrong image. I did however blot the layers with white powder.

I used a number of different owl references to create the desired effect. (Having looked at the final piece the two areas of improvement I could have made would have been to strengthen up the face and add more feathers to the forehead and cheeks.)

Egyptian goddess

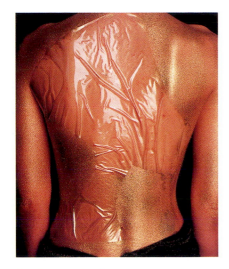

1 Plastic is placed across the back to make a stencil and gold is airbrushed around the stencil.

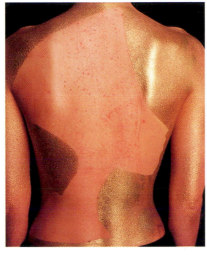

2 The plastic is removed.

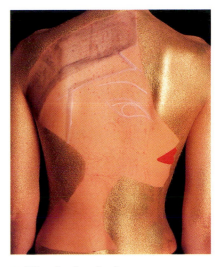

3 The design is drawn.

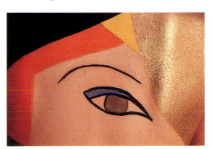

4 Detail of paint work.

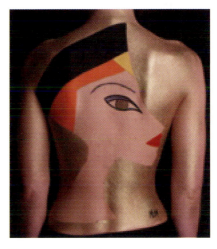

5 Finished look.

Make-up artist
Marie de la Motte

Airbrushing

Airbrushing became popular in the 1980s, particularly for fashion effects. It is now enjoying a revival in the American film, TV and beauty markets and slowly filtering through to Europe. However, the finished look is at times too perfect for most work. Used mainly in fantasy special effects and body painting, it gives a clearer, fresher blend and coverage than the sponge and brush method. Airbrushing is invaluable for covering large areas quickly and evenly and can replace coloured sprays used in hair work. It delivers a much finer film of colour, giving a perfect graduation from light to dark, and is particularly effective when using stencils. There are two types of airbrush available:

1   The airbrush that works with an electric compressor: these are available in different shapes and sizes with silencers, fans and extra knob fittings. The airbrushes have different storage facilities for the make-up. Some have a small well on top of the brush for smaller areas. Some have small jars that attach to the

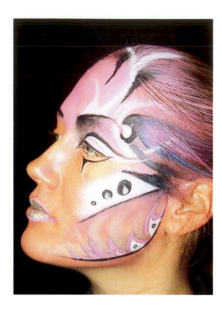

bottom of the airbrush to contain the make-up; these are good for covering larger areas. Some have both attachments.

2   Also available are the smaller more portable kits in which the airbrush propellant comes in the form of a gas can. These are less expensive in outlay, but the cost of the gas cans adds up if used regularly.

Both types are capable of airbrushing but the compressor set-up can achieve a more detailed effect – though much more expensive and less portable. Airbrushing equipment can be bought from all good professional make-up and artist suppliers. The watercolour body paints are available from professional make-up suppliers.

A word of warning to everyone when airbrushing. It is important to have good ventilation in the room you are working in and to take every precaution to protect yourself and the model from inhaling airborne paint vapour. Without a ventilating fan or open windows, airbrushing is definitely a health hazard. This applies particularly if a number of people are airbrushing at the same time in a confined space.

Airbrushing is used not only for fantasy effects but also for painting large areas swiftly, such as contouring shadows on a human body or dummy. It is also useful for a final finish to tie a look together on top of brushwork and sponged effects. For a fast, even-coloured background, the airbrush can give a good paint finish with hand-painted detail on top. It is excellent for spraying hair instead of aerosol can sprays and can produce perfect looking lines when sprayed against masked off areas.

Depending on the dexterity of the artist, airbrushing can add a slick 'fresh from the factory' look. Students are advised to attend a course to learn the basics of cleaning and maintenance of airbrushes, the different pressures of air flow and the different strokes used to create various effects. The art of airbrush application provides another useful tool for the make-up artist's repertoire of skills.

Step-by-step

The Golden Girl

This make-up was inspired by the golden girl in the credit sequence of the film *Gold Finger* and a Madonna music video.

1   First the model was painted gold using a sponge and liquid gold body make-up.

2   Then a plastic stencil was used to outline the design (plastic supplied by the roll with adhesive backing available from good stationery shops).

3   Red liquid body paint was airbrushed across the stencil and peeled off when dry to prevent the paint from 'bleeding'.

4   The nails were painted black.

5   The hair was backcombed and airbrushed gold to match the body.

6   The make-up was based on a fashion look with red smoky eyes (using eyeshadow). The lips were covered with vaseline mixed with glitter.

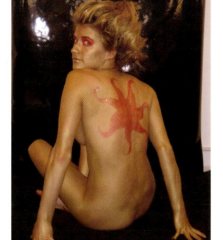

Make-up artist Cecilia Blomstedt

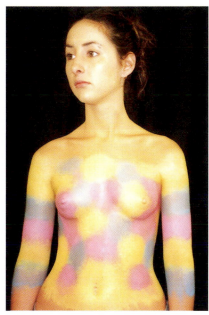

Trying out the design on a
dummy

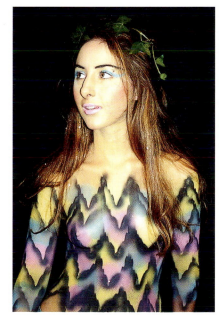

Creating the base

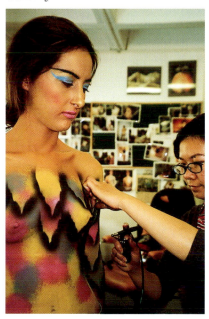

Using a leaf as a stencil to
create the repeat pattern

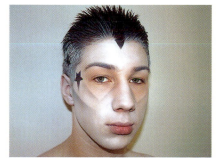

The finished look

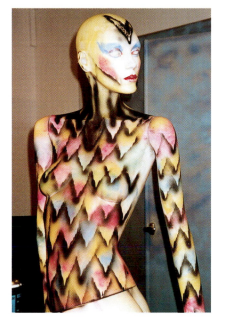

Airbrushing detail with stencil

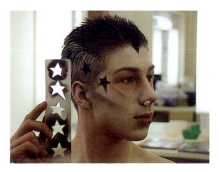

Finished effect

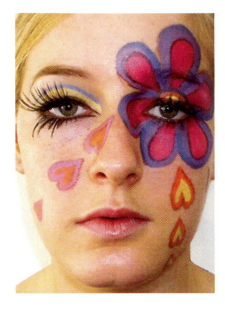

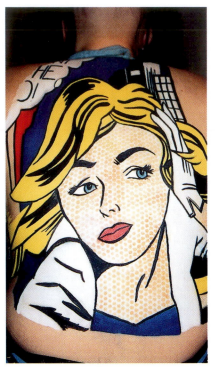

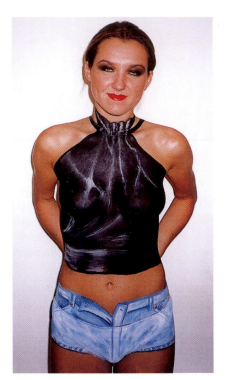

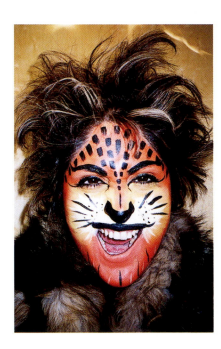

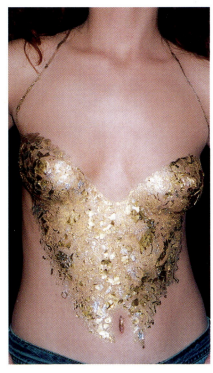

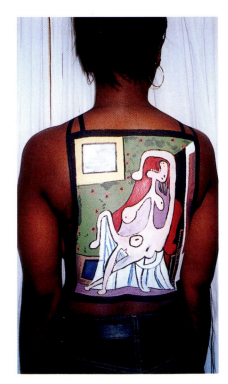

Face and body make-up by students of the Delamar Academy

Working in theatre

5

Introduction

The history of theatre dates back to ancient times as the earliest form of entertainment. It has evolved through Shakespeare and music hall to the spectacular, sophisticated form of stagecraft today. It has been under threat of television, but despite technology has remained popular. It seems that, no matter how far computer special effects advance, there is no substitute for watching actors, singers and dancers perform in front of us. It is the purest most disciplined craft of all – and employs dedicated, creative people.

To work in theatre, the make-up artist must have knowledge and experience of working with wigs and facial hair. This aspect of the work is extremely important. In fact the person in charge of the make-up and hair is known as the wigmaster or mistress. Stage make-up has become more realistic looking over the years. The traditional style of heavy lines, sometimes crudely applied, is no longer used. Current thinking is that even in large auditoriums the make-up should be suitable for the audience sitting in the front rows (stalls) because they pay the most for their tickets. Another reason is that the performance may be recorded for television transmission. This happens regularly in the Royal Opera Company, where the 'in house' make-up artists work full time on all the various productions being performed throughout the season.

Many make-up artists with hair skills begin their careers working in the theatre, usually as wig dressers, employed on a casual basis. The performers generally do their own make-up, but the make-up artists help them if necessary and always organise the quick changes. Special make-up effects such as making and applying bald caps or wounds and blood are the responsibility of the hair and make-up department. In addition they do all the hair work, including making wigs and facial hair on large productions.

One of the most exciting aspects of working in theatre is that it is 'live'. Each performance is unique and the excitement generated by an appreciative audience creates a buzz which is only experienced in this area of entertainment. Timekeeping, self-discipline and team spirit are essential for the performance to work as a whole.

The hair and make-up designer is responsible to the show's overall designer, which is unique to the theatre. After the designer has decided on the 'look' of the sets, costume, lighting, hair and make-up, the heads of those departments work out how to apply and maintain the required effect, taking into account the practical needs such as quick changes, health and hygiene, etc.

Once the style and method of working have been established, it is important to stick rigidly to the routine for reasons of continuity and for the sake of the actors' confidence. If the show goes on tour to different venues in other countries, the formula must remain the same. If local make-up artists are employed on tour, they will be shown the make-up to be used, how the wigs are set and every detail of the quick changes. Sometimes there are only two or three minutes to change an actor's costume, hair and make-up back stage. The make-up artist has to stand in the same spot at precisely the same time for each performance and change the wig or make-up exactly the same way each time. This is very important, since the show must be identical wherever it is performing.

Another important aspect of make-up for the theatre is that it has to last without touch-ups throughout the entire scene. Whether dancing, singing or fight scenes, the wigs must not fall off and the make-up must not run. Sometimes this may pose a problem. For example, if the dancers have to change from one look to another, it may be easier to remove water-based make-up more quickly than oil-based greasepaint or creams. But watercolours are tricky because they run when dancers sweat. Powder make-up might be considered an easier alternative, but powder can cause dancers to slip if it gets on the floor or on their feet, so the safety of the cast would be a priority. The hair and make-up designer has to address many such decisions before the final rehearsal.

For anyone wishing to work in this area it is best to gain work experience in small theatres and amateur productions, learning as much as possible. After that, attend a good training course which covers all the different facets of make-up and hair (particularly wig dressing) before approaching large theatres in the capital cities. The head of hair and make-up in the particular theatre should be approached. If given an appointment, the trainee should present their portfolio and ask for work experience or to be hired as a casual worker. A little knowledge or interest in that particular theatre or its current productions would help the head of department to recognise the person as enthusiastic. Most trainees start this way and once the door is open they often find a niche in this most rewarding area of show business.

Case Profile
Pam Orange, Hair and make-up manager

How long have you been working in the industry?

I have been working in the theatre industry for over 17 years. I worked part-time as a hairdresser while the children were growing up, but once they had grown up I decided I wanted a career.

How did you get into it?

I secured a position as a part-time wig assistant at Opera North in Leeds, and after a while I was taken on as a full-time assistant. I watched and learnt from Peter Owen, who was one of the leading wig and make-up designers in film. Shortly afterwards I became head of hair and make-up at Opera North.

After 4 years I left Opera North to become a supervisor at the English National Opera based at the London Coliseum (ENO). Within a few years I became head of the wig and make-up department which involved running shows and supervising production at the company workshops. The company was under the direction of Peter Jonas along with David Poutney and Mark Elder.

After six years I left the ENO to go freelance. Since then I have done musicals, dance, plays, more opera and many varied projects. In addition I have been involved with teaching students at the Make-Up Centre in London, and I have toured extensively in the UK and abroad.

What or who has been your most significant project?

I became hair and make-up supervisor for a dance company called Adventures in Motion Pictures (AMP), where I worked on *Swan Lake*. It was my first experience of working in dance. After London the show went on to Los Angeles, on its first major foreign tour. By the time we reached LA I had it running like a military operation. *Swan Lake* later went to Broadway and then followed a tour taking in numerous cities throughout the world. Wherever the show went it got the same reaction full houses and lots of cheering, people loved it. I felt privileged to work on it.

I have been with AMP for more than five years now as head of hair and make-up, but *Swan Lake* will stay with me forever as the most exciting, enjoyable and challenging project I have ever done.

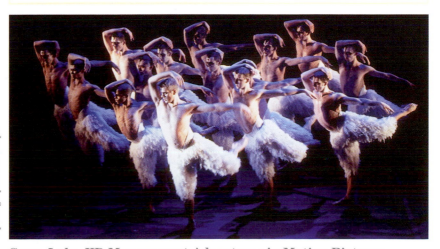

© photographer Bill Cooper

Swan Lake, **KD Management Adventures in Motion Pictures. Make-up artist Pam Orange**

What do you enjoy most about your work?

I enjoy production weeks when a show transfers from rehearsal room into the theatre: seeing the set for the first time, bringing together artists in new costumes and wigs and meeting with props, wardrobe, lighting and stage crew. I like unpacking, getting settled in a new room and shopping for stock plus finding the way to the stage and generally getting used to the layout of a new theatre.

Even a production that you know very well has to be adapted, especially during a tour when we move from theatre to theatre. I am constantly thinking of new ways to make the transition from dressing room to stage or quick-change area as easy and as stress free as possible. I like transferring ideas into something practical and workable, while always keeping within a budget. Most of all I enjoy being part of a team and the hands-on creative work that is involved in perfecting the show, the buzz of a live audience and passing on my skills to the next generation of hair and make-up artists.

What advice would you give to people trying to get into this area of work now?

You have to be able to work as part of a team; it takes 100 per cent commitment every night from everyone to produce a show. Be prepared to change and adapt and think quickly.

If this is for you, be prepared to take on anything at first, watch from the wings, listen and learn. As the saying goes 'you are only as good as your last job' so do it well. Every task, no matter how small, makes a show and moves you forward in your career.

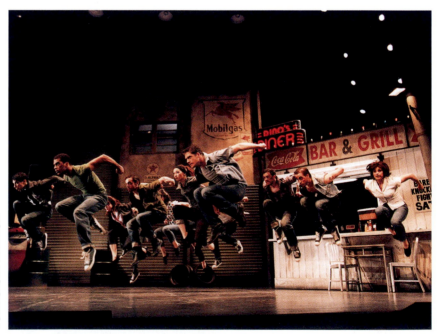

© photographer Bill Cooper

The Car Man, **Adventures in Motion Pictures.**
Make-up artist Pam Orange. Producing director Katherine Dore.
Designer Lez Brotherstone. Directed and choreographed by
Matthew Bourne.

Make-up for small and large auditoriums

In intimate theatre there is often no need for the actors to wear strong make-up, especially if the play is set in modern times. Stylistic effects with too much make-up look old fashioned when the audience is close to the actors, and many female performers apply normal street make-up most of the time. In the smaller theatre companies and for amateur productions, the actors look after their own appearance. They are usually very appreciative of help with their make-up if approached by students, particularly when wigs and facial hair are involved. To judge the results of your work, it is best to observe from the point of view of the audience during a full rehearsal, when the lights have been set. Notes should be taken on every actor's make-up and hair in order to make final adjustments if needed.

In the larger auditoriums such as the Royal Opera House, the Coliseum or the Olivier stage at the Royal National Theatre, the make-up is viewed from a longer distance than in intimate theatre. Theatres such as these have full-time make-up artists who hire or make the wigs and are responsible for maintaining the hair, together with the make-up and any special effects. For such large auditoriums the make-up may be stronger because of the distance from the audience. Sometimes a freelance make-up artist may be contracted to design the make-up for the entire cast, and to then teach the performers to apply the make-up themselves. This has occurred on many long-running musicals and the make-up artist might be called in every so often to revamp the look if it seems 'tired'. On *Phantom of the Opera* a make-up artist was engaged full time to apply the prosthetics piece for the phantom make-up and a freelance prosthetic expert provided a regular supply of prosthetic 'masks' so there was a new one for every performance.

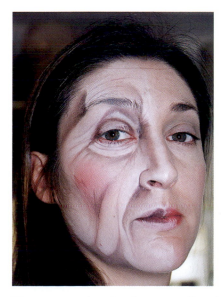
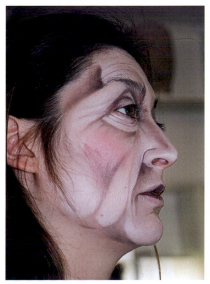
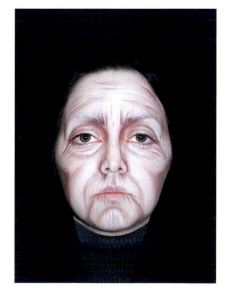

Theatre ageing for large auditoriums
Make-up Trefor Proud, Hollywood Academy Oscar winner 2000

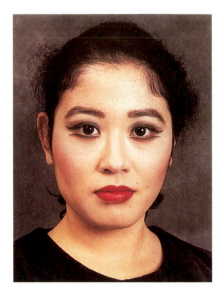

A straight theatrical make-up: strong eyelines are used and red is blended under the bottom eyeline to enhance the eye from a long distance

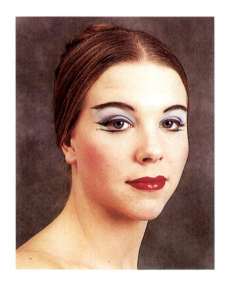

Make-up for the ballet

Basic principles

The main considerations when doing make-up for the theatre are the *distance* involved and the *colours* normally used in theatrical lights; usually these are cold colours in the blue and green range. The principle followed in dealing with the distance is to make up the face *strongly* and *cleanly* using the basic corrective make-up techniques: strongly because both the strength of light and the distance will reduce the impact of the make-up; cleanly because otherwise the facial definition will fail to register at a distance.

To deal with the lighting, the face is made up in warmer tones than usual, with emphasis on the red and orange tones and on certain areas of the face.

Planning the make-up

Make-up for the stage should not be heavy or overdone. The foundation can be as lightly applied as for TV and film. What matters is that the right colours and shades are applied in the correct places so as to give definition to the face.

In a large auditorium only a small proportion of people will be able to distinguish the make-up. For those seated further away from the stage, the actors' faces will be a blur. As you can't meet the needs of everyone, it is best to apply make-up that will look believable to the front section of the house. The middle to last back rows will simply view it as part of the overall picture of performance, costume, lighting and wigs.

In general, the make-up for actresses on the stage should include stronger eye make-up than would be normal for film or TV, darker or brighter lipstick and a stronger colour on the cheeks. Bear in mind, however, that although the colours should be stronger, the placing must be exact and the blending subtle. Avoid hard lines – the eyelines, for example, must always fade to nothing at the ends. The amount of make-up used and the application should be as light as for any other area of the media.

Ballet make-up

Make-up for the ballet traditionally comprises very pale skin tones, whitened shoulders and arms and strong eye make-up.

Effects of theatre lighting on make-up

The lighting is usually set at a 45–degree angle to the stage and must counteract any shadows. *Overhead lighting* is also used: these lights are changed and operated during the production. *Colour gels* such as 'mid-sapphire blue' are used over the lights. These 'bleach'

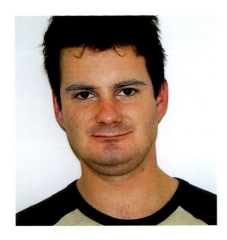

the make-up and drain colour from the faces, so more red and warm colours have to be used in the make-up. Lighting changes the make-up colours:

- White make-up looks blue, so cream should be used
- Blue make-up looks black, so use brown
- Yellow make-up looks washed-out white, so use reds, oranges and pinks

Prior to the opening night there is a full *dress rehearsal*. This is the time when the make-up artist can check the make-up from the audience's point of view. Any shadows that need correcting can be checked, as can the strength of the colours used in the make-ups.

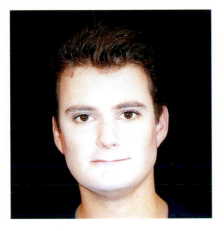
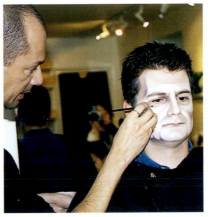
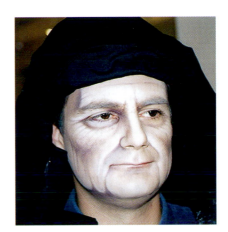

Ageing for opera
Make-up artist Trefor Proud.
Hollywood Academy Oscar
winner 2000

Case Profile

Caroline O'Connor, Wig assistant and make-up artist

How long have you been in the industry?

I completed my course in July 1999 and have been very fortunate as I have been working consistently since January 2001. I started as an assistant on *Swan Lake* at the Dominion Theatre and was then offered a position on the *Lion King*. During this time I was promoted to make-up artist and responsible for a couple of principal make-ups. I decided to expand my experience and am currently a wig assistant on the *Sunset Boulevard* tour where I am learning a lot about wig dressing.

How did you get into it?

I had always wanted to be a make-up artist and I also had a great interest in the theatre. I used to volunteer to be the make-up artist for many local amateur dramatics societies. During this time I had been working in a very high-pressure sales environment and once I reached my thirtieth birthday I realised that I was very unhappy with my job and felt unfulfilled. After a lot of consideration I decided to take the plunge and obtained a loan to go to the Delamar Academy and train to become a make-up artist. This turned out to be the best decision I have ever made. I love my work and have never looked back.

What or who has been your most significant project?

The *Lion King* was a very special time for me as the production is very respected and it taught me a great amount about what is expected of a make-up artist and the pressures that can come with it. The costumes, puppets and set, as well as the make-up and wigs, are a visual feast and to be part of that was a great privilege.

What do you enjoy most about your work?

I enjoy learning on new projects and with each new project comes further experience and confidence. It is a wonderful feeling when you put make-up or a wig on an artist and it looks fantastic. Their appreciation and enthusiasm for your work is very rewarding. On a practical note, I enjoy working in the theatre as the hours suit me and it is also very social in the evenings – especially on tour!!

And least?

Working in the theatre is very repetitive as your cues each day very rarely alter. It can be quite tough as there is very little variety in your day-to-day structure and this can be a little disheartening, especially on a matinee day when you have two shows.

What advice would you give to people trying to get into this area of work now?

Pinpoint shows that require your skills and find the name of the Head of Department. You may find that there are no positions available at that time, especially if a show is current so you need to be persistent. It maybe an idea to offer holiday cover or ask for work experience. This way you have a chance to show your enthusiasm, which is so important especially at the beginning of your career. Once you have a position, take your sense of humour with you and leave your troubles at home as a cheery personality goes a long way!

Modelling with wax

Sometimes modelling a feature with light and shade is not dramatic enough and a three-dimensional effect is needed. In such circumstances *putty* or *wax* can be used to change the shape; **mortician's wax** is generally used for this purpose. The wax is covered with a special liquid *sealer* and allowed to dry. It can then be made up to blend with the rest of the face.

Nose shapes

Although wax may be used anywhere on the face, it is generally most successful in changing a nose shape. A very small amount can product a striking change in appearance and does not hinder an actor's ability to speak. However, if used too far up between the eyes, the wax will lift and look unnatural when the actor smiles or

Equipment and materials

- wax
- artist's modelling tools (wooden and metal)
- water
- powder
- moisturiser
- sealer
- camouflage make-up or a grease-based palette
- foundation
- various make-up materials for the finished result
- isopropyl alcohol (to clean the brush when using sealer)

frowns. It should therefore start below the bridge of the nose and blend naturally at the edges to a thin consistency.

Wax is tricky to use, but modelling becomes easier with practice. Keep your hands cool and dry or the wax will become too sticky to work with, rather like making pastry.

Method

Stage 1

1 Make sure that the skin is grease and oil free.
2 Apply a thin coat of wax to the nose, as a base for further application.
3 Soften a small ball of wax with the fingers.
4 Mould a rough shape and apply it to the nose. Work cleanly – keep your hands cool to prevent the fingers from becoming too sticky. (Dip your fingers into a bowl of cold water from time to time.)
5 Use a modelling tool to blend the edges so that the join is invisible.
6 Work up and out from the natural bone and nose shape. Don't work up the bridge of the nose (between the eyes): wax here would wrinkle with any natural movement.
7 Build width, keeping a contoured shape without ridges.
8 With a modelling tool or your fingers, blend the wax into the natural shadows and folds of the real nose. Work quickly and positively. For the best result, use the minimum wax.
9 When you are satisfied with the shape, use your fingertips to smooth a little moisturiser or cleansing milk onto the surface to keep the wax smooth and remove any tackiness. Use the tip of your finger to smooth away any imperfections.
10 Apply texture, if needed, using a rough towel, orange peel or a stipple sponge. This will give an open-pored look.
11 Apply a thin coat of **sealer** with a brush. Allow this to dry.
12 Apply a second thin coat of sealer with a brush. Again, allow this to dry.
13 Apply a third thin coat of sealer. This time, tap a little translucent powder onto the surface while it is still tacky. This will prevent any shine from the sealer and wax showing through the make-up. Use a soft mop brush loaded with powder, tapping the stem of the brush so that the powder drops onto the sealer, making it matt.

Stage 2

When the top coat of sealer is dry, make-up and colour pigmentation should be put on top to make the wax look like living flesh. Be sure to match the surrounding skin tones.

14 Study the colours and tones of the surrounding skin on the face.
15 Make a mental note of any other pigmentation marks, such as freckles, broken veins or redness.

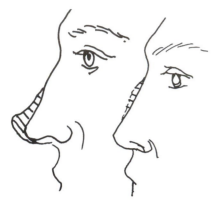

Nose shapes

16 Camouflage make-up provides good coverage, or you can use your normal grease palette. Use a soft sponge or brush to apply rose, pink or red to the wax; be careful not to dent the wax. Use more pink and red than you would imagine necessary. This is to give the effect of blood flowing beneath the surface. Wax always appears too pale on camera, paler than it does to the naked eye.

17 Powder gently, using a soft brush; then apply some yellow and brown colour with a soft sponge. Powder again.

18 Apply foundation colour all over the face in the usual way and be careful when applying it on top of the wax nose. Check that the nose blends in naturally with the rest of the skin tone.

19 Powder the face and apply the rest of the make-up according to the required style.

When the entire make-up is complete, check the nose. Make sure that the shape is rounded and natural looking from all angles. A little more wax can be added to hide any imperfections. Remember to add colour tones, base and powder to any extra application of wax.

Tip

● When applying foundation to wax noses, it is helpful to add a little moisturiser: this makes it more pliable, and easier to spread.

● When stippling on pink and red colours, remember that the wax is opaque: it will take plenty of colour to match the skin tone.

Changing the shape of a nose using wax

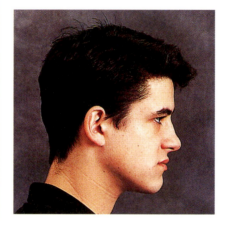

Before

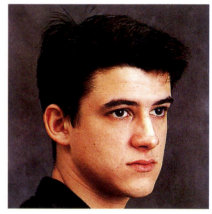

A small amount of wax has been applied

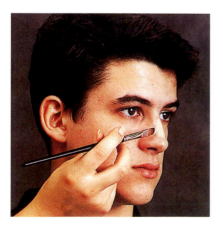

Blending the edges with a modelling tool

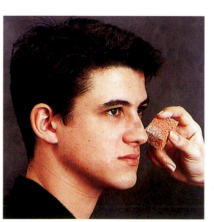

Applying colour to match the surrounding skin tone

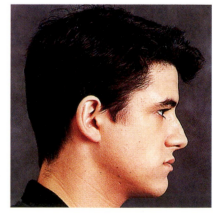

Foundation and powder have been applied for the finished effect

In warm weather, the wax will become very soft and sticky. Keep dipping your fingers in cold water to prevent stickiness. Throughout the make-up, wipe tools regularly with isopropyl alcohol. Clean the brush used in applying the sealer by keeping it in isopropyl alcohol.

Guidelines

Before you start, study the nose you are going to change and choose a shape that will look natural. If the face is small, do not plan a huge nose as this would look false.

Don't use too much wax – if you do it will be harder to shape and blend. Take care in modelling the wax or it will look like a stuck-on blob.

Avoid blending the wax onto the cheeks: it is much harder to hide the edges there. Confine the work to the bridge of the nose.

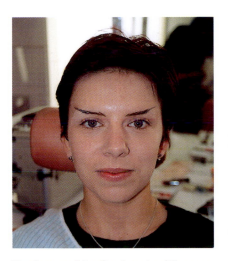

Eyebrows blocked out with wax and redrawn

Theatre work

For stage work it is usual to apply a layer of spirit gum to the natural nose before applying the wax. This prevents the wax nosepiece from falling off during the performance! When the gum is tacky, a small amount of cottonwool can be used as a bond. The wax is placed on top and modelled in the usual way.

Other uses for wax

Wax can be used to build up any area of the face provided that there is not too much movement of the underlying muscles. The most effective places are bony areas such as the cheekbones, the chin and the forehead.

Blocking out eyebrows

Wax is very useful for blocking out – **waxing out** – eyebrows, as for an eighteenth-century period make-up. Before applying the wax, use a bar of soap to flatten down the natural eyebrows. This will prevent the hairs from poking through the wax.

1   Wet the end of the soap bar and use it to flatten the eyebrows firmly to the skin.

2   When the soap has dried, use a modelling tool or spatula to apply a thin layer of wax on top of the soap.

3   Seal the wax using one or two applications, allowing each layer to dry.

Tip

When drawing eyebrows on wax, use a *ruler* to make sure that the brows are evenly matched. It is surprisingly difficult to get both eyebrows the same if you are not following the natural brow bones.

4   Colour the wax with make-up and apply foundation colour to the entire face. Make sure that the eyebrow areas match the foundation colour.

5   Paint in the new eyebrows with brush and greasepaint. (Pencils are not successful on wax as they are too sharp.)

Blocking out the eyebrows

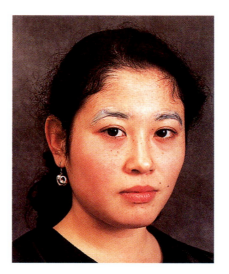

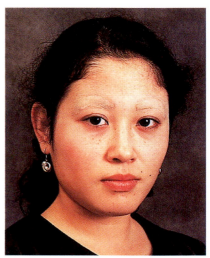

Eyebrows have been pressed down with soap to flatten them; wax is smoothed on top with a modelling tool. A sealer is painted on top of the wax

When the sealer is dry, camouflage make-up is used on top and the whole face is ready to be made up

Working in television and cinematography

6

Introduction

Television

In the 1950s and early 1960s, television was transmitted in black and white. With the advent of colour in 1967, the make-up changed completely. Hair work became more important. Switches and other hairpieces were added to dress long, swept-up styles such as the 'beehive'. Eyelashes were worn by most women – full sets of lashes above and below the eyes or individual lashes painstakingly applied one by one.

Working in black and white, we had thought simply in terms of black, white and shades of grey. With colour, the whole concept of make-up changed, but it was a gradual process. Although we worked towards colour, not many people had colour televisions, so most continued to watch the programmes in black and white. Everyone on the production team had to undergo tests for colour blindness.

As colour became more common in all transmissions, skin tones suddenly became more important. It was first most noticeable when making up politicians and news announcers. For black and white we used to powder down a politician to eliminate too much shine or to tone down a heavy beardline. In glorious colour, however, every red nose or flushed face was noticeable. If a government minister had had a drink or two in the hospitality room before a TV appearance, this would be obvious to the viewers at home. More time and care was needed if make-up artists were to offset such problems. From then on we had to pay attention to the elimination of redness and the addition of warmth through blushers and eyeshadows.

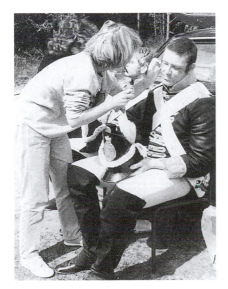

Working on location

Case Profile
Kevin Fortune, Make-up and hair designer

How long have you been in the industry?

I worked in Customs and Excise at Heathrow airport, but decided that I wanted a job with a little less aggression, more creativity and much more travel involved. I took early severance pay to take a course at the Delamar Academy.

How did you get into it?

When I finished my course, I worked in bars and clubs so I could work for virtually nothing on any programme or test shoot during the day. I was desperate to work within fashion and ideally I wanted to work with famous models. Fashion shoots were few and far between. After a short spell of no work, I focused on TV and was soon inundated with assignments. That was the big turning point in my career.

What or who has been your most significant project?

I am experienced in all areas of make up and have worked on many programmes and films. My first film was *SW9* shot in Brixton, it included beauty make-up, drug addicts, complex scars and specific wounds, all-over body tattoos, a human statue with body painting and two complex wigs which with the help of make up artist Jo Evans, we made ourselves during filming. The whole job was very demanding and challenged me in every way. It covered everything I could think of and I loved it.

What do you enjoy most about your work?

I always have and always will greatly enjoy everything that I do. Life is 365 days a year.

And least?

The only aspect that I am not keen on is paperwork, and Pop videos are not at all glamorous. Very long hours, lots of sitting around, very loud music early in the morning. This is a career choice that I made. It's all good and even when it's bad, it's still good.

What advice would you give to people trying to get into this area of work now?

You need an ability to understand human behaviour and the capability to adapt to new circumstances and not to take on board other people's problems. Working for a cosmetic company gives you the opportunity to gain in depth knowledge about make-up and skin care. The fastest way to learn what does and does not work on individual faces was through individual customers. Also never to turn down unpaid work, as people usually return the favour.

My most important point is to believe in yourself, have faith in your artistic talent and know that you will be very successful. There will be a time when your ability is challenged but there is always a way through to make you stronger and more efficient.

A career in television make-up

The most important aspect of working in television is to be able to work as part of a team. There is no room for histrionics behind the camera. Make-up artists must be tactful, diplomatic and remain quietly in the background. Much emphasis is rightly laid on this aspect of a make-up artist's job, because very often you are the last person to speak to the performer before he or she appears in front of the camera. The make-up room should therefore be an oasis of peace while everywhere else in the studio is hectic.

It is important that you work fast, but it is also important that you remain calm. There should be no sense of panic. It can sometimes be hard to maintain calm confidence when an assistant is hovering nearby asking 'How much longer will you be?' or warning 'You've got three minutes'. (It is the floor assistant's job to make sure that the performer is *on set* – that is, ready and on the studio floor – by a certain time.)

Like every other industry, television has changed and will continue to do so. All make-up artists must be geared to the *freelance* world and its uncertainties and trained in the different areas of make-up in order to be able to make a successful living: the training needs to address the demands of the industry. A freelancer has to work across the board, to be good at everything, including both make-up and hair. If you have a flair for certain areas of make-up, such as fantasy or prosthetics, that's fine, but recognise that not as many jobs require these skills as, say, wig dressing, straight make-up or ageing. You are therefore wise to gain experience in all aspects of make-up, even if one day you hope to specialise in a particular area.

It still takes five years to become confident and worthy of the title make-up artist. The work experience during these first five years will help to form the type of make-up artist you become. Freelancing is highly competitive and you need to be of the highest standard if you are to succeed. The more you learn, the more there is to discover. Explore new techniques, be willing to learn from more experienced colleagues and never imagine that you know it all. When you become confident in the make-up field, start learning from other departments about lighting, camera and costume.

Make-up offers a truly fascinating career in television. You meet talented, interesting people; friendships form, and the feeling grows that you belong to a team – a team that, in a remote location, becomes your family.

These are real aspects of make-up work and they are good, but do not be misled into seeing this career as glamorous. If, for example, you find it hard to get up at 4 am or to work all night, don't become a make-up artist. The hours are both long and unsocial. When working on a TV film there is no time at all for a social life. Six-day weeks have become normal in the industry and you may be required to go anywhere in the world. As well as warm, sunny locations this can include cold, damp places. Standing in the freezing cold in some isolated place at 6 am is not everyone's idea of good working conditions. Long hours and long absences from home impose real strain on relationships with partners. Often the make-up artist is the first person to start work in the morning and the last to go home at night. Above all, you need to be strong and healthy because you will never be able to take time off with a simple cold. The show must go on!

Working on location

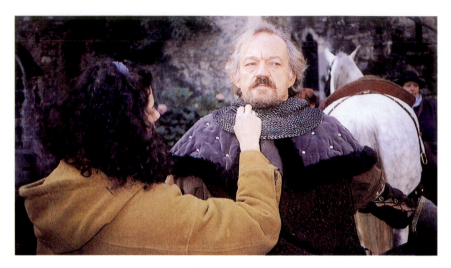

Case Profile
Jane Fox, Make-up artist

How long have you been working in the industry?
Since 1963.

How did you get into it?
I did a beauty course after leaving school. Whilst working in a salon, I met a TV make-up artist. She put the seed in my mind. I applied for a job as a trainee make-up artist at ABC Television and was taken on at their Manchester Studios. We did a lot of light entertainment shows. In those days of black and white television the make-up was heavy and very orange. I then spent several years working in the States. When I returned, the switch to colour meant lots of new skills to learn.

What or who has been your most significant project?
My seven years at the BBC, doing a lot of period drama productions, were a highlight. I loved doing the research and creating the appropriate hair styles. Afterwards, when I'd left the Beeb and was freelancing, it was great fun because of the variety of work. I met lots of new people and worked with many different production companies on films, TV, pop promos and commercials. Those were good days, which also fitted in with having a young family.

What do you most enjoy about your work?
I love life on the set, the company, the sociability – the idea that I'm contributing, and needed. Painting faces is a particular thrill, especially that moment when I see the transformation take place before my eyes!

And least?
The early starts, now that I am working permanently on a 24-hour News channel.

What advice would you give to people trying to get into area of work now?
I'm now in a position where I interview new make-up staff. Chiefly, I'd say, you need to be able to do a make-up within a time limit and to get on with other people. This means creating a good atmosphere in the make-up room and on set. Be prepared for long and unsociable hours and very early starts. Always work hard and be willing to help and learn. Other key qualifications for a job in TV (as in other media) are good hairdressing skills, imagination, creativity and a clean, up-to date, well-stocked kit.

Assistant or trainee make-up artist

When working as an assistant to the make-up designer, it is important that you listen carefully and carry out instructions. She will have already designed the look of the make-up and hair for all the actors, including the one you have been assigned to look after.

Trainees and assistants should always be flexible and willing to change their approach to suit the needs of the make-up designer. Some designers will give you a free hand and allow you to use your own initiative, especially when they know your standard of work. Others will give specific instructions and even notes or charts on the individual actor's requirements.

It is always a good idea to 'chart' the make-ups you are doing when working on a long series or film. If you became ill, someone would have to take your place, maybe at an hour's notice. No one is indispensable, of course, but it is very difficult to take over a make-up from another artist and achieve exactly the same look without the aid of written notes, sketches or Polaroid photos.

When making up for crowd scenes – the background people known as *extras* or *crowd artists* – it is not necessary to make notes about the individual faces you make up. Here you will work towards a general look, depending on the period: for the 1940s, for example, appropriate hairstyles, matt red lips and emphasised eyebrows with pale skin tones for the women; short haircuts, moustaches and no beards for the men. The make-up designer will issue instructions and the assistants must interpret them and carry them out.

Continuity is important in television and it is up to every make-up artist to maintain continuity in her hair and make-up work. As an assistant, then, there is plenty to do. You may be left on the set **standing by**, ready to retouch the make-up if necessary. Be sure not to leave without permission from the designer. If the director calls for make-up, there should always be someone from the make-up department within view and earshot. In summary, your job is to support and assist the make-up designer – to be a responsible, reliable and active member of the make-up team.

Senior assistant make-up artist

The senior assistant make-up artist also should provide back-up for the designer. Having had years more experience than a trainee make-up assistant, she will be given the more important or difficult make-ups to do, usually for the principal actors who will have the most close-ups. She will also have such responsibilities as the designer chooses to give her – paperwork, shopping, attending wig fittings or contacting suppliers by telephone. This is because in the absence of the designer she would have to be able to take decisions. Whilst working as a chief assistant, she is really training to become a designer herself.

Make-up designer

The make-up designer is responsible for the make-up *budget* allowed. Within this budget she must plan and organise everything: how many wigs; which stock to purchase; how many assistants to hire; the entire look of the hair and make-up.

After some weeks or days in preparation, including planning meetings with the rest of the key crew members – the director, costume designer, set designer and so on – she will aim to be ready for anything needed on the shoot. She will have *broken down the script*, contacted the actors, arranged wig fittings and sent scripts to her chosen assistants. By the time the crew has assembled to start filming, the make-up designer should have organised everything. Make-up materials will have been purchased, tests carried out if necessary, wig and facial hair fitted and dressed and transport and accommodation arranged with the production office.

This *pre-production work* can be a difficult period, especially if time is short. Actors may not have been cast until the last minute and there may be a frantic rush to get everything done. If the director changes her or his mind about something, rearrangement may be necessary at the last minute. The designer is responsible to the director for whatever look is required. Interpreting the director's wishes is not always easy as many do not know what they want until they see it. Yet whatever the director may ask for, if it relates to the make-up or the hair, it is the make-up designer's job to produce it somehow.

For special effects, such as artificial features (*prosthetics*), the make-up designer will contact a specialist, hiring out the work if the budget can meet the expense. If not, she will make the piece herself, with the help of assistants. It is for the designer to judge which is the most sensible option, basing her decision on the assignment, the circumstances and the budget.

The designer should also look after her assistants, making sure their working conditions are up to standard, with adequate lights, mirrors, space to work, sleeping accommodation, regular meal breaks and so on. She should encourage and instruct any trainees, building up their confidence. At the same time, she must keep a supervising eye on all that is going on, remain in touch with the production office, take any new instructions from the director and make up the leading actors.

In television, each person should know exactly what his or her role is in the overall scheme. A highly professional TV crew working well together on the studio floor is a fine sight. Not every team will gel together, but at its best, with the combination of technical expertise and professional grace, it can seem like a well-choreographed ballet. To be a part of something like that, when it happens, is a remarkable and wonderful experience.

Developing the designs

Having first read the script, the make-up artist should attend a preliminary meeting with the producer, director and costume designer to discuss the interpretation of the script and the *style* of the production. The make-up artist then researches the style of the production, using books, old photographs, magazines, videos, old films and the like. If there are special requirements, such as make-up for illnesses, burns or wounds, the make-up artist may need to consult medical experts or police records. Having completed the research, the make-up artist begins to make plans:

1   She **breaks down the script**, marking items needing her attention (e.g. when a character needs a 'wound with running blood')
2   She *lists* the number of characters and *walk-ons* (extras, or crowd artists) involved
3   She *compiles* a *cost breakdown* for the producer
4   She discusses this with the producer and agrees the *budget*
5   She contacts the artists, through their agents or the production office, to discuss the 'look' required and to determine whether wigs, facial hair or prosthetics are needed.

A more detailed breakdown of the script must be made to choreograph any make-up changes during filming. This is done in consultation with the director and the costume designer so that everyone is working to a common end. This is vital if continuity is to be maintained when scenes are shot out of sequence. The actors will also want to discuss their ideas. When everything has been taken into consideration, the make-up artist will be ready to design the make-up and hair.

Providing sketches

Drawing the idea on paper is the best form of communication: one sketch can save hours of talking. The drawings can be passed on to the various specialists, to show precisely how the wigs, facial hair or prosthetics should look. Once the design is on paper, it must be approved by everyone involved. This includes the director, the actors and the producer and – in the case of wigs, facial hair and prosthetics – the specialist makers.

The initial design is a starting point, which can be discussed and modified where appropriate. The final design, once agreed, can be photocopied and distributed to the wigmaker, the facial-hair maker or the prosthetics expert, as necessary. The design element in make-up is present throughout the make-up artist's work. Despite this ideal procedure, in practice many make-ups are designed directly onto the actor's face, if time does not allow pre-production sketching.

If there is enough time for planning the schedule and breaking down the script, that time is well spent in thinking through the entire project. After the research, perhaps relating to an idea

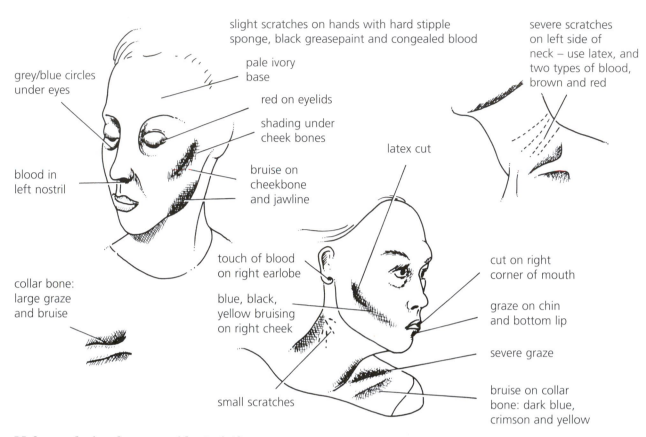

grey/blue circles under eyes

slight scratches on hands with hard stipple sponge, black greasepaint and congealed blood

pale ivory base

red on eyelids

shading under cheek bones

severe scratches on left side of neck – use latex, and two types of blood, brown and red

blood in left nostril

bruise on cheekbone and jawline

latex cut

collar bone: large graze and bruise

touch of blood on right earlobe

blue, black, yellow bruising on right cheek

cut on right corner of mouth

graze on chin and bottom lip

severe graze

bruise on collar bone: dark blue, crimson and yellow

small scratches

Make-up design for an accident victim

already at the back of your mind, the intended result should be captured on paper where it can be improved until it seems to work well.

Sketches should be well presented, with additional notes and instructions as necessary to help those involved to achieve your concept. Copies can then be sent to the specialists where postiche or

Make-up designed for Sir Anthony Hopkins as 'King Lear'

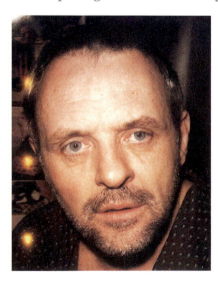

A Polaroid of the actor

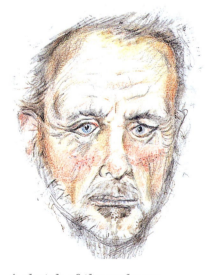

A sketch of the make-up

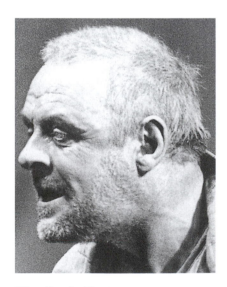

The final effect

A make-up record chart

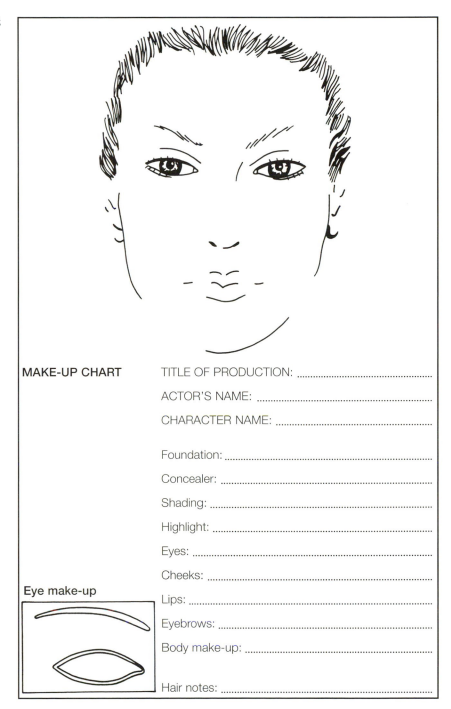

MAKE-UP CHART

TITLE OF PRODUCTION: ....

ACTOR'S NAME: ....

CHARACTER NAME: ....

Foundation: ....

Concealer: ....

Shading: ....

Highlight: ....

Eyes: ....

Cheeks: ....

Eye make-up

Lips: ....

Eyebrows: ....

Body make-up: ....

Hair notes: ....

prosthetic pieces need to be made. It is a good idea to cover the drawing with a layer of tracing paper. This will protect the artwork and prevent it from getting dirty. Notes and comments can be written on the top layer of greaseproof paper.

Make-up and hair designs can range from a simple chart with written explanatory notes to a detailed drawing filled in with colour. One method of working out the design is to use a photograph of the actor, drawing the face on paper and then superimposing the design on top. This is a good way of working out the shape of a nose or how the face might be successfully aged with make-up.

Continuity

In film and television the scenes are shot out of sequence for numerous reasons – perhaps because the locations are the priority, or perhaps the actor has only four weeks to finish his scenes before starting another job. In effect it means that you could be working on the last shot of the film involving actors continuing a scene that was shot a year ago. In fact it is quite normal for a film to be finished and for scenes to be re-shot unexpectedly when the producer decides to do so. The crew members, including the make-up department, may be working on other productions by then so new people are hired to film the pick-up shots. Watching the film played back, notes on the continuity at the time are essential. Obviously the actors must be dressed the same, have the same skin tones, hair length and colour and the same make-up or everyone will notice when the film is edited together.

For example, if the producer of a television soap series decides to do some pick-up shots of close-ups of the actors from scenes shot four months previously, the make-up artist may have to solve a number of continuity problems:

- wardrobe matching the clothes since many of the costumes may have been hired and returned to the hire companies
- matching the hair: various hair pieces may need tracking down, as some may have been hired and returned to the wig makers
- matching the make-up: foundations, lipsticks, eyeshadows and blusher may have been used up or lost

Whilst such scenarios can be stressful at times, they are all part of the job. In feature films there is a *script supervisor* who deals with the general continuity of the filming, type of film stock, camera lenses used and dialogue changes.

It is still up to the individual departments to work out their own continuity, by taking Polaroids or digital photographs of all the main actors – front, back and profile views – as well as notes. All changes of hairstyles, costume and make-up should be logged with the scene number and day number of the film sequence.

To make life easier, a make-up artist will keep a hairstyle the same shape. When the action of the filming calls for the hair to be wet or untidy, photos must be taken. The action may take place in a rain storm exterior which might have to match up to the actor walking into an interior with wet hair. The interior scene might be shot in the studio months later and must match up to the exterior shot. Make-up and hair artists often have to apply beards and moustaches to match an actor's natural facial hair which he subsequently shaved away, or supply a wig because the actress has had her hair cut short. Continuity is very important in television and filmmaking.

Make-up and hair continuity

Linda A. Morton is currently the make-up designer on *Night and Day*, Granada Television, which is a multi-episodic soap on ITV. Here, in her own words, she provides an insight into some of the techniques she has developed for make-up and hair continuity.

Make-up and hair continuity for television and film is crucial. It does not matter how good you are at your make-up skill, if your continuity is incorrect the viewer's attention will be distracted from the story.

To date most of the work I have been involved with has tended to be multi-episodic drama for television, but the same theory that applies to TV also applies to film. Multi-episodic means that instead of having one story, like a film, you have multiple episodes. This is like lots of short, contained stories all muddled up together. As you can imagine, making sure that the actors have bruises in the right places and on the correct scenes has to be planned out in advance so no errors are made. When productions issue their filming schedules, the scenes are all out of sequence, which could be due to a number of reasons such as an actors' availability or location availability, etc.

Try to imagine your first day filming. You might shoot scene 1 of the story and then the next scene you film that day might be the last scene of the story, scene 30. If your actor got beaten up in a fight in a bar in scene 29, you know that by the time you film scene 30 your actor should be bruised. Therefore you would need to plan a make-up change for the second scene of the day to make your actor look as if he's been beaten up. This is how I start my breakdowns.

A story day

Story days are like days of the week: Monday would be story day one, Tuesday story day two, Wednesday story day three, Thursday story day four and Friday story day five. Imagine the following scenario in a film or television show:

- A man gets up on Monday morning (story day one) and on his way to work he is mugged and gets a black eye
- Tuesday (story day two) the black eye would be a real shiner
- Wednesday (story day three) it's getting better
- Thursday (story day four) it's much better
- Friday (story day five) it's nearly gone

If you think how the black eye would change from a make-up point of view, it would be a bad black eye and then slowly getting better. Read the next part on character breakdowns and you'll understand how to keep track of the changing make-up in television and film.

Character breakdowns

When I break down my character sheets, I try to keep it simple. In the following scenario, there are three different make-ups:

A character sheet

Linda A Morton
Make-up Continuity Character Sheets

Film: Episode No:

Actors Name: Scene No:

Characters Name: Story Day:

Direct Continuity To:

PHOTO: HAIR NOTES:

MAKE-UP NOTES:

- Make-up A is a day make-up
- Make-up B is a party make-up
- Make-up C is a bed make-up

The scenario, which could occur in a soap, is as follows: A woman gets up out of bed (scene 1). She takes a shower (scene 2). Immediately after her shower she goes into the kitchen to make breakfast. During breakfast she has a conversation with her mum (scene 3). After breakfast she dries her hair, gets dressed and puts on her make up to go to work. She goes to work (scene 4). That night she goes on a date. Later she arrives at the restaurant for the date and she has put her hair up and changed her lipstick (scene 5). Let's break down this scenario.

Scene 1

In the first part of the scenario – scene 1, where she is getting out of bed – I would make that actor up as Make-up C (i.e. a no make-up look) because she has just got out of bed. I would fill out my character sheets *Make-up C*. For every character sheet you need to fill in the scene number and story day. Under make-up notes you need to fill in what make-up you used to create that look so that you could recreate it if the scene needed to be reshot. This is also the reason why you need to take a photo on set on the good take (i.e. the take they will use on the programme or film).

This information should be included on the character sheet

Under make-up notes I'd add:
MAC C3 foundation
YSL Touche Eclait
MAC C3 Studio Fix Powder
Waterproof mascara (n.b. There is a reason for using waterproof mascara – she will have a shower in Scene 2, your actress will have lovely lashes in the shower that won't smudge!)

Under hair notes I'd add:
Hair messy (just got out of bed) used Paul Mitchell Hair Wax.

Scene 2

She has a shower in scene 2. Now this is a different make-up. It's still Make-up C, but she now has wet hair so I would fill in another character sheet including that information. Again you need to fill in what scene and story day it is. In this instance, the make-up notes would remain the same. Remember, we thought ahead – our actress does not have smudged mascara in the shower she looks nice and fresh faced. The only real difference (apart from the scene number and of course the photograph) is that hair notes would now read 'Wet hair (is in the shower)'.

Scene 3

In scene 3 she is making breakfast and chatting to her mum. It's still Make-up C and she still has wet hair. Don't forget to fill in another character sheet with the same information as the previous one but the correct scene and what story day.

Scene 4

In scene 4 she's dried her hair and now she is putting on her make-up. It's now Make-up A (day make up) and she is going to the office so she would be smart and neat. That information should reflect in what style of day make-up you do.

This time, I'd include the following information on the character sheet:

Under make-up notes I'd add:
MAC C3 Foundation
YSL Touche Eclait
MAC C3 Studio Fix Powder
Shu Uemura silver eye shadow
Black coal eyeliner under eye
Bobby Brown Plumb Blush
Collection 2000 nude lipgloss
Waterproof mascara

Under hair notes I'd add:
Hair half-up and neat brown clasp.

Tip

A helpful hint when you take your Polaroid: make sure the actor is aware that you are about to take their photograph and *always* announce clearly just before you take the photo. You don't want to blind unsuspecting actors with your camera flash! Warning them that their photo is being taken will avoid this.

Scene 5

She's arrived at the restaurant in scene 5. It's now Make-up B (party make-up). All she's done to change her look for her date is put her hair up (in a French plait) and changed her lipstick, but you need to do a character sheet with that relevant information. Don't forget to fill in the scene and story day.

Always take a Polaroid of the actor on set after they have rehearsed and started filming. Listen out for the first assistant director or the director indicating that it is a 'good take' or 'print it'! This means that it is the piece of footage which they will use in the finished television show or film. Only take your Polaroid on the good take, otherwise you do not have a correct photograph of the continuity of that scene – and it's also a waste of film.

Breaking down the schedule

You normally get a *schedule* at the start of the job from which to do your preparation. The scenes on the schedule will be muddled up and out of sequence. In addition to the schedule, you should also get the *scenes in story order*, which is the schedule in scene/story order and a *character and scene list*, which is a list of the scenes that individual characters are in. This information comes from production who get it from the Movie Magic Scheduling Programme.

I start with the character and scene list. Don't worry it looks more complicated than it is! I use one page per actor for the continuity breakdown sheet, filling in the character name and the actor name at the top. I copy from the character and scene list what scenes the actor is in and I fill in the scene numbers in the left-hand column on the *continuity breakdown*. I would then look up in the *schedule in story order* the first scene that the actor is in on the top of the page that I have just filled in of the continuity breakdown. I would then fill in the remaining information, time of day, story day and the location.

Take one actor at a time, from their continuity breakdown sheet look up the first scene in the script that the actor is in and read it. You then decide if they are Make-up A, B or C and fill in that information under special make-up/hair on their continuity breakdown. Remember to look out for the story days!

Continue this way throughout the script paying particular attention to stage directions like 'she has been crying' or 'his black eye looks really sore'. If, for example, an actor was crying in scene 6, time of day 10 pm, it's story day one and she is in the bedroom and her make-up is A, you have filled out your character sheets noting Make-up A and she was crying (haven't you?!!!). So when you come to film scene 7 which is only 10 minutes later in the story (remember you might film this scene three weeks after you have filmed scene 6), you will know from your notes that she had been crying in the previous scene and therefore maybe smudged mascara or some tears from the top of scene 7.

Once you have finished your breakdowns you can then put the information in a folder. Having broken down the whole script, you know what you are doing in every scene. All you have to do now is film it!

A continuity breakdown

Continuity Breakdown						
Character:				Artist:		
Sc	Time	Day	Location	Special Make-up/Hair	Details of Scene	F

Call sheet breakdown

A call sheet is what you get every night informing you of what scenes will be filmed the next day. I have made a template which is an 'at a glance view' of what Make-up A, B or C you will be doing on your actor that morning.

First, you fill out on the call sheet breakdown what episode, scene and story day you will be filming that day from the call sheet. Then you fill in from the call sheet what actors are in each scene (on the first line).

Next you look up your notes from your continuity breakdown folder and fill in if it's Make up A, B or C and any relevant notes, for example, is crying underneath their name (on the second line). Now if it is the first day of filming and no one is established, then you will also fill in your character sheets and establish your characters.

At the end of your filming day you file your actors' character sheets with their photographs stuck onto them into folders all ready to copy again exactly if you are filming scenes of the same story day and the same make-up. The key to good make-up and hair continuity is to be organised, diligent and always aware of what is going on around you!

A call sheet breakdown

Linda A Morton			Call Sheet Breakdown			Make-up Department			
EP									
SC									
SD									
EP									
SC									
SD									
EP									
SC									
SD									
EP									
SC									
SD									
EP									
SC									
SD									
EP									
SC									
SD									
EP									
SC									
SD									
EP									
SC									
SD									

Example continuity sheet from *Night and Day*   **NIGHTANDAY**

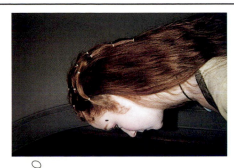

Holly
66B/20
69C

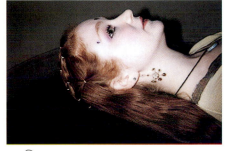

Holly
66B/20
69C

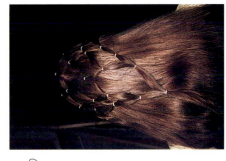

Holly
66B/20
69C

Linda A Morton
Make-up Continuity

Film:

Episode No: *66B*

Actors Name: *Phoebe Thomas*

Scene No: *20*

Characters Name: *Holly Curran*

Story Day: *69C*

Direct Continuity To:

HAIR NOTES:

Director has requested lattice hairstyles

PHOTO:

Holly
66B/20
69C

△ fardel

* pink glow

MAKE-UP NOTES:
Base Clinique
Touche under eyes
Studio fix
Eyes – fardel over lid
Mac – pink glow
Grafite liner + under
Black mascara
3 false eyelashes under
Pink glow
Lips – pink poodle

Case Profile
Linda A. Morton, TV and film make-up artist

How and when did you start in the business?

I joined the Harlequin Theatre Group which took me as a trainee in their wig Department. This led to other theatre groups and in 1993 I took a make-up training course.

Was there a turning point in your career?

When *Lock, Stock and Two Smoking Barrels* was released it led to other jobs, including *Taggart*, *Dream Team*, and *Night and Day*.

What do you consider to be important qualities for a make-up artist?

Good humour, patience with actors and assistant directors and, of course, the skills in the job.

How has your career changed your life?

I've made great friends and achieved goals that I never thought I would, especially when I think back to amateur theatre days.

What have been your most satisfying jobs?

Lock Stock and Two Smoking Barrels, I have great memories from that film. When it was released in the cinema my family were very proud.

What advice would you give to young people entering the industry?

Keep trying! Be the best work experience placement that the department has had make tea, clean brushes and work surfaces, do the laundry, etc. Work on student films and learn all you can from them. Also be punctual, it gives a good impression.

Do you think the TV/film/theatre world is glamorous?

It is glamorous – lights, camera, action, all the sparkle and excitement of launch parties and premieres. I have though worked on *Taggart* in the pouring rain and gale-force winds and sleet even that was fun.

What would you consider to be the best and worst aspects of being a make-up artist?

The best is doing a job that I love and working with my friends. The worst is the unsociable hours.

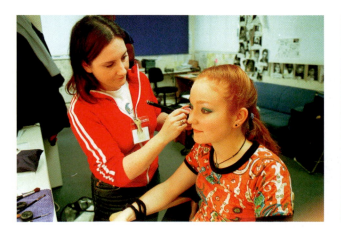

Linda Morton working on *Night and Day*, a Granada Television production

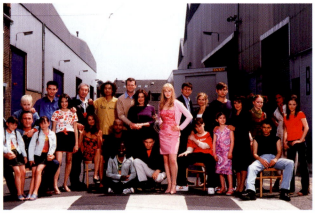

The cast of *Night and Day*, a Granada Television production

Case Profile
Leda Shawyer, Make-up artist

How and when did you start in the business?

I started in 1997, after graduating from university. Having spent three years doing academic work, I wanted to do something creative so I took a course at the Delamar Academy of Make-up.

Was there a turning point in your career?

My turning point was meeting make-up designers who then took me onto jobs with them.

What do you consider to be important qualities for a make-up artist?

You need enthusiasm, patience, a sense of humour, to have a good rapport with people and you need to be artistic.

How has your career changed your life?

I have met fantastic and interesting people, made some very good friends, had lots of fun, and filmed in places I would never normally visit.

What have been your most satisfying jobs?

I find doing make-up other than the usual 'straight' make-up most satisfying. On *Topsy Turvy* I learnt much about theatre make-up and facial hair, and *Band of Brothers* involved dirtying down soldiers and creating wounds and special effects.

What advice would you give to young people entering the industry?

Be keen and enthusiastic and be prepared to do anything.

Do you think the TV/film/theatre world is glamorous?

People think TV and film work is glamorous, but the reality is long hours, sometimes standing all day in mud and rain, usually in very unglamorous locations.

What would you consider to be the best and worst aspects of being a make-up artist?

The best aspect of being a make-up artist is meeting great people, and doing a fun creative job; each day is unpredictable. The worst aspect is long unsociable hours.

Leda Shawyer making up Honor Fraser on *The Cookie Thief* (a short film)

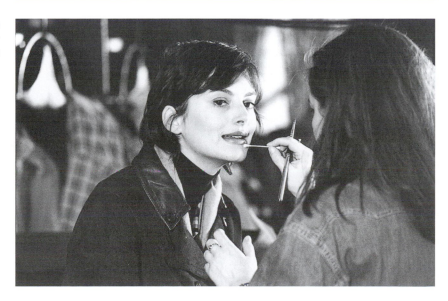

Cinematography

Working in cinematography

Cinematography is the most expensive, high profile, artistic form of product in the entertainment industry. The history of film making goes back a long way – before television was invented. Cine films, or moving pictures taken with a cine camera, were flickering black and white silent films featuring actors who swiftly become known as movie stars. The vaudeville houses were closing and the motion picture industry was building film palaces.

Once sound was added to films, the actors' voices were as important as their looks. A new cast of movie stars appeared in the 'talkies' and the old favourites of silent film quickly lost favour if they had squeaky voices. One of the stars of vaudeville, Mae West, successfully transferred to films. By the mid-1930s the child star, Shirley Temple, was awarded a special Academy award. Mae West, some 40 years older, paid more tax than any other woman in the USA. Soon there were glamorous women such as Greta Garbo, Ingrid Bergman and Betty Grable to represent the alluring faces of cinematography.

Films were made for propaganda during World War Two (1939–45) and the Korean War a few years later. A favourite post-war classic *Casablanca*, epitomises the individual heroism, sacrifice and romantic yearning of the era. Starring Humphrey Bogart and Ingrid Bergman, the film provides excellent research for the make-up and hair of the wartime 1940s look. By 1947 the film industry was expanding in England as well as the USA. Twenty studios were in full production in and around London and looking for personnel to train.

The film studios in 1947

The film studios included: MGM (Elstree), ABC (Elstree), Brit. Nat (Elstree), The Gate Studio (Elstree), Danziger Studios (Elstree), Pinewood Studios (Rank), Denham Studios (Rank), London Film British Lion (Shepperton Studios), Gaumont Studios (Hammersmith), Islington Studios (London), Warner Bros Studios (Teddington), Twickenham Studios, Wembley Studios, Bushy Studios, Ealing Studios, Bray Studios, Merton Park Studios.

Case Profile
Tom Smith, Make-up artist

The directors with whom Tom Smith worked dominated the film industry in the second half of the twentieth century. Tom's credits as a Chief Make-up Artist include *Charge of the Light Brigade*, *Raiders of the Lost Ark*, *Indiana Jones and the Temple of Doom*, *The Shining*, *Ghandi* and *Gulliver's Travels*. He has worked with many directors including Laurence Olivier, Orson Welles, Alfred Hitchcock, Richard Attenborough, Stanley Kubrick and Steven Spielberg.

How long have you been in the industry?

Since 1947.

How did you get into it?

I tried to get a job in the art department at Pinewood studios, but they had no vacancies. The art director took me to the make-up department who were looking for people to train.

I had no wish to be a make-up artist but I soon found myself really sucked into the scheme of things. In the afternoons I worked in the small laboratory in the make-up department – modelling, casting and making prosthetics. I was fortunate to be put on a salary from the first day.

What material was used in prosthetics in those days?

In those days we used thermal plastics to represent flesh.

Was there much work being done with FX then?

At that time the only make-up artists interested in prosthetics were Stuart Freeborn at Pinewood and Charlie Parker at MGM Elstree. The methods developed by these two remain the same today – the perfect material to put into the moulds hasn't been found.

You have so many wonderful stories about these people. What was your most memorable project?

I'd say in the early years working as an assistant to Stuart Freeborn, Charlie Parker and Toni Sforrzini. As an assistant I had a free hand, I was concerned only with what I did. As chief make-up artist you were concerned not only with what you were doing, but also what was going on in the other make-up rooms.

What make-up brands did you use in those days?

In 1947 the main supplier was Max Factor. For black and white films you used Panchromatic foundation bases ranging from 1–31 (orange in colour). The female base, normally no. 6, would be two shades lighter than the male, which was usually no. 8. This was irrespective of the part you were playing, so the maid got the same base colour as her mistress and the refuse collector got the same base as his lordship.

Everyone had to be made up. For colour productions, Max Factor sold a special make-up base for Technicolour, ranging from 1–12. The same principle of the men being slightly darker than the females still applied. Then Max Factor brought out a range called N series (from 0–12). The N stood for Neutral. This could be used for either black and white or colour.

The advent of colour must have changed everything for make-up artists. How did you adjust to the advance of technology?

Improvements were being made with cameras and film stock all the time. For example, when cameramen developed the use of effect lighting for colour, as they had for black and white, make-up artists had to adjust and develop their own style.

The unions were very strong in those days. Could you work without being a member of the union?

You could only work in the studios if you held a union card. For make-up you had to be a member of NATKE (one of the three film unions). The other two were ATC and ETU. To be a member of NATKE you had to be selected for training. You trained for 6 months without pay and then took a test. If you passed the test you were in, and could register at the NATKE employment office, as available for work. You could only take the test once, so if you failed you were out.

What advice would you give to people starting today?

Well you would think that they should have some schooling in art but this is not necessarily the case. Charlie Parker was into sculpting so he spent a lot of time modelling. Stuart Freeborn didn't come from that background, he was always practising make-up as a kid. He had thousands of pictures of make-ups on himself. The point is that you have to want to do it to start with.

You should start modelling in clay, learning to use your hands. Observe faces, and study paintings. Rembrandt's self portraits at different times in his life say it all. You could do ageing or character make-up the way he paints, breaking up the face, avoiding lines. I use blobby bits of brushwork in the same way – putting in shading and highlights.

Students should get into painting on paper as well as modelling in clay. Get used to working with colours and then try it on a real face – working their way with that.

Then you have to get on with people. The job isn't just about putting on make-up, its also about getting the actors in front of the camera in a good frame of mind so that they can work. You have to be flexible, do what they want to begin with to win their confidence. For example, you couldn't tell Liz Taylor that you didn't like the black stuff around her eyes. That's how she saw herself because someone had sold it to her. So you had to win her confidence, win her over. Don't be adamant about things – you need a bit of charm. At the same time keep your dignity. You need to handle people gently but firmly. Sometimes you are asked to do things that seem impossible.

Can you give an example?

When working with Basil Dearden [the Director] on *Gordon of Khartoum* we used the Egyptian Camel Corps as guards. Basil wanted all the men in the Camel Corps (all Nubians with blue-black skin tones) to look white. Basil's chauffeur was Nubian, so I got him into a guard's uniform, with the headgear with feathers, etc., and tried out different colours on him. I used reds, pinks, yellows, and different colours to avoid that chalky, ghost-like look you get on blue-black skin tones when you add pale colours. I made him up, all except his hands and put on a reddish blond moustache. Then I took him in full costume to show Basil, who looked at him and said 'yes, so what?' I showed the man's hands and he realised then and said, 'Oh my God – that's great.' He said he wanted them all done like that. There were two to three hundred of them, so I said I would need two to three hundred make-up artists to get them done quickly. In the end Bill Lodge, John Webber, myself and six Egyptian make-up men did it with pancakes, putting in plenty of reds and warm colours. Of course they couldn't be seen in close ups. But it worked all right.

On the first *Indiana Jones* film by Steven Spielberg 1981 you decided to have Harrison Ford with a three day beard growth. This started the designer stubble look, which was fashionable all through the 1980s and 1990s. What gave you the idea?

Oh, I just wanted to make his face look a little more interesting, really. You need to be a Jack of all trades and a master of everything. It all comes with experience. You can tell students everything, but you can't give experience. It depends on how much they listen, how intense they are about their work.

The role of the film make-up artist

The key make-up and hair artists, sometimes called designers, are responsible for the research, design and execution of make-up and hair on all major film productions. They must choose and supervise all members of the make-up and hair departments allocated to the production, making sure that the required style is achieved on all artists.

They must liase with the producer, director, costume designer and actors to decide the style of the film, whether it be modern day, futuristic, realistic, fantasy, stylish, period, down market, etc. They also work in close consultation with the director of lighting and the set designer. They must be available for planning meetings at any time.

The make-up and hair budgets are the responsibility of the key make-up and hair artists/designers, also called heads of departments (HODs). The make-up HOD is responsible for the designing and ordering of wigs. There will usually be a separate department for prosthetics if required on the film.

The prosthetic HOD liaises with make-up, hair and all other departments previously mentioned. The make-up and hair HODs should be involved at the earliest stages of the production. Sometimes it is even necessary to be involved in the decision of casting an actor, particularly if prosthetics and special effects are to be used. There is a great deal of work to be done prior to filming. This is known as pre-production planning and preparation. The first stage is to read the script.

Pre-production planning

First meeting

Having read the script, the make-up and hair designers attend a preliminary meeting with the producer, director and costume designer, to discuss the interpretation of the script and style of the film.

Research

The make-up and hair designers then research the style of the production, using books, old photographs, videos, old films, magazines, etc. to help with the work.

Script breakdown

The make-up and hair designers break down the script, listing the number of characters and crowd artists involved.

Cost breakdown

They then do a cost breakdown for the producer, which is discussed and a budget is agreed. The budget will include the number of staff required, make-up materials, etc.

Contacting the actors

The make-up and hair designers proceed to contact the actors, through their agents or the production office, to discuss the character and the look required and whether they will need wigs, facial hair, contact lenses or prosthetics.

More script breakdown

A more detailed breakdown of the script has to be done in order to choreograph any changes. This is usually carried out in consultation with the designer and costume designer, so that continuity is maintained when scenes are shot out of sequence. All the other departments go through the same procedures so that everyone is working to a common end.

Employing staff

The make-up and hair designers now contact their choice of make-up artists to work with them on the film. These would usually be an experienced senior make-up and hair artist each, sometimes called a supervisor, who would be a continuity assistant. The supervisor also helps with further script breakdowns, makes appointments for facial hair and wig fittings and generally backs up their HOD in all preparations. On large-scale productions three or four extra make-up and hair artists might be booked.

Dental work and contact lenses

The make-up department is responsible for making appointments for actors when special dental technicians are needed.

If **contact lenses** are required, the make-up designers must work in close consultation with the optician, deciding the colour and shape of the lenses and arranging fittings for the actor.

Working on location and checking facilities

The make-up and hair designers consult with the location manager in order to make sure that proper facilities are available to do the make-up and hair, for example, a Winnebago caravan equipped with proper lighting, running water, adequate space, power points, etc.

Final fittings

Arrangements are made with the wig makers and prosthetics department for final fittings. Any actors who need hair cuts, colouring or styling are taken to a specialist hairdresser, or else the hair department do them if time allows. For period productions the crowd artists will have facial hair fitted and labelled individually by the make-up department whilst haircuts or wig fittings are the responsibility of the hair department. This is often done two or three days before the first day of filming.

Wigs, facial hair and prosthetics

The HODs are responsible for the collection or delivery of wigs, facial hair and prosthetics.

Lighting tests

Prior to the commencement of filming, the director of photography (DOP) will arrange for a lighting test and the principal actors can be seen in costume, with make-up and hair or any special effects. This gives the director a chance to prove the finished look or discuss changes.

Organising the make-up rooms

The make-up and hair departments organise their individual rooms based at the studio or, if going on location, supervise the loading of all equipment to be taken to the arranged place. *Pre-production planning is now finished*.

Production filming

The make-up, hair and costume HODs arrange with the assistant director (AD) the times for each individual make-up, hair and wardrobe call for the actors. The AD works out a schedule which fits in with the general shooting schedule. These are all posted or given out by 4 or 5 pm the previous day.

The key make-up artist/HOD/designer designates which of his/her team of make-up artists looks after which actor, giving detailed notes and reference pictures if necessary. The key make-up artist also makes up the main actor and takes total responsibility for all make-up done on the production. The same applies to hair and costume departments. All continuity is the responsibility of the HODs, helped by the rest of the make-up and hair personnel, using Polaroid and digital cameras, notes and sketches.

After filming

On completion of shooting, the make-up and hair designers are responsible for checking and returning all hired wigs, completing paperwork involved in the production and doing a budget breakdown of all monies spent to be sent to the producer and accounts department.

Case Profile
Christine Blundell, Make-up and hair design

In 2000 Christine Blundell and Trefor Proud were awarded Oscars by the Academy of Motion Pictures Arts and Sciences for the make-up and hair on *Topsy Turvy*, a Mike Leigh film. They were the youngest ever winners in the category of make-up and hair.

Shortly afterwards Chris was awarded a BAFTA in Britain. For a make-up artist this is a dream come true. Here Christine Blundell explains in her own words how she researched the period, a vital part of the preparation process prior to filming, and shows some photographs of the actors as they appeared in the film.

How long have you been in the industry?
Fifteen years.

How did you get into it?
Initially I started 22 years ago as a hairdresser working in London doing lots of hair shows and promoting hair extensions in the early 1980s. I opened my own salon and then sold up after a few years and invested the money into a make-up course.

What or who has been your most significant project?
Topsy Turvy is by far the most significant project, having been told by Mike Leigh, the director, over a year before we started what his idea was. The 'designers' of the film were: Eve Stuart, set design; Lindy Hemming, costume; myself as make-up and hair designer. We sat down and had a constructive chat in which we concluded that, since Mike is renowned for his real, tell-it-how-it-is films, if any little thing we did was not periodically correct we would indeed be hauled over hot coals by the press. So the research began.

Anyone familiar with Mike's work will know that there is no script, so theatre wigs, hair pieces and transformations (an add-on fringe that fastens at the back of the head – Queen Mary loved them!) were all made exactly as they were at the time, hand stitched inside or out, so they could be used as a prop or to wear. Also the theatre chorister wigs were made as a job lot and the wigs of the principal theatre stars – the Three Little Maids – were made with no expense spared! This was probably what happened at the time and what still happens.

The make-up on the theatrical side was strictly only the colours of greasepaint they had at the time. We had the luxury of having our extra help make-up people for a few days, to teach them the now quite primitive method of application. For our everyday principal actors who were not in the theatre slap, any facial hair was hand laid into existing facial hair to 'bush' it out. The female principals were good enough to let us use burnt cork as eye definer/mascara and a lip/blush colour that I'd had made up from a remnant of a colour I'd found.

The company Charles Fox was brilliant and allowed me to access its archives. I even got hold of one of Charles Fox's original books on theatre make-up at the time. All in all it was a wonderful project – made even better by resulting in an Oscar and BAFTA for me and an Oscar for my assistant, Trefor Proud. He truly deserved his award for his incredible knowledge of theatre history and countless other make-up talents.

This shows that research in our line of work can be incredibly enjoyable and much more interesting for me than any history lesson ever was. Although pulling off something like, say, a quick effect on screen might have taken weeks to sort out, it's worth it when it works.

What do you enjoy least about your work?
Long hours and early mornings have to be the worst part and not being able to throw sickies if you don't feel up to working that day.

Chris Blundell doing make-up
on Timothy Spall for the film
Topsy Turvy (Oscar winner,
2000)

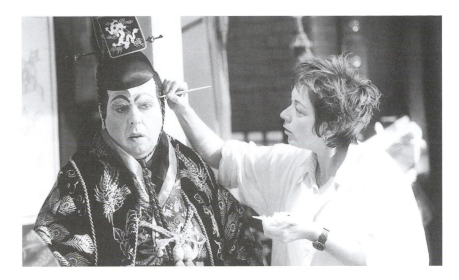

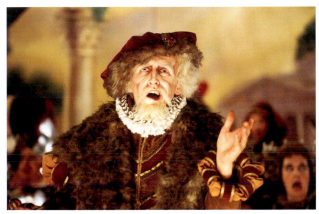

Actor: Martin Savage

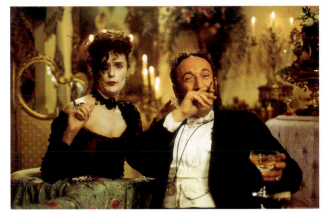

Actors: Katrin Cartlidge and Allan Corduner

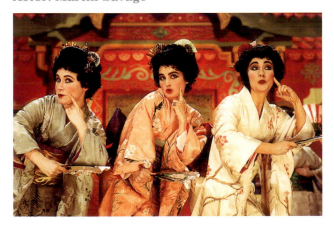

'Three Little Maids'. Left to right:
Cathy Sara, Shirley Henderson and Dorothy
Atkinson

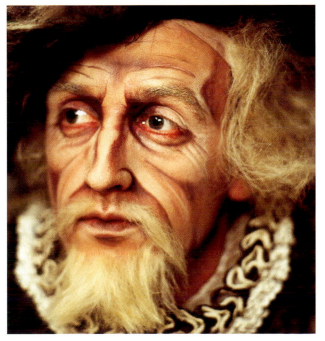

Topsy Turvy
Make-up Chris Blundell. Photograph Simon Mein

Close-up of Martin Savage. Make-up by Trefor
Proud

Who does what on a film

Title	Responsibilities
Producer, associate producer, executive producer, producers' assistants	All handle the business side of the film. They are the money people.
Production manager	Works for the producer, responsible for the daily running of the production.
Assistant director (first AD)	First assistant director responsible for the shooting of the film. He assists the director and commands the set. Calls 'action' and 'make-up checks', etc.
Second and third assistant directors	Training to be producers or directors. Responsible for cast and crew to be in the right place ready for shooting at the right time. Responsible for make-up/hair, department's schedules.
Editor	He edits the film together with the director.
Musical director	Responsible for the music on the sound track.
Camera crew	
Director of photography (DOP) or cinematographer	Responsible for all that is seen on the film.
Camera operator	Operates the camera and does the camera work.
Assistant camera (or focus puller)	Responsible for the focus and reloading of the camera.
Stage or set crew	
Gaffer	Chief electrician in charge of setting up the lights for the DOP.
Best boy	The gaffer's assistant.
Electricians (or sparks)	Responsible for moving and changing the lights.
Key grip	Responsible for moving the camera, laying tracks for the tracking shots.
Props	They place the furniture on set for the designer.
Set dresser	They dress the set and are responsible for the look, as directed by the designer.
Designer	Responsible for the building of sets, locations and overall look of the film.
Design assistant	Assists the designer.
Sound recordist	In charge of the sound, operates the sound equipment.
Boom operator	Holds the boom near the actors to record the sound and assists the recordist.
Sound supervisor	Responsible for the overall continuity, working closely with the director and noting which shots he/she wants to keep and where he wants to cut the film.
Director	Has complete charge of the action of the film, the cast and crew.
Casting director	Finds the right actors for the parts.
Stand in	Someone with the same height and build as the star actor who stands in while the lights are set for the film.
Doubles	Someone who doubles for an actor when the distance is so far that you wouldn't know the difference.
Stunt double	Someone who does dangerous things that an actor doesn't do.

Title	Responsibilities
The cast	
Stars	The principal actors whose names appear above the title of the film.
Featured actors	Well-known actors in supporting roles.
Crowd actors	Non-speaking, or make crowd noises.
Make-up and Hair Artists	Responsible for all the make-up and hair needs of the entire cast, plus the doubles and stunt doubles.

On small budget films the make-up and hair are often done by the same person, particularly if the needs are simple. On major feature films it has always been the custom to have two separate departments for make-up and hair. The standard of excellence required for work which is shown on a big screen means that more personnel are needed for a good result. Very often a star will have his/her own choice of make-up artist and hair stylist.

Case Profile
Lois Burwell, Make-up artist

How long have you been working in the industry?
Since 1979.

What or who has been your most significant project?
Many projects were significant in a variety of ways. If I had to choose one film probably *Mona Lisa* because it began a series of films, which became the foundation of my career. So thank you to Neil Jordan for taking a risk with a relatively unknown make-up artist. In recent times it would have to be *Braveheart*. The reasons span from the personal to the professional. The work was challenging and I met my husband, plus it gave me the honour of an Academy Award, which was a wish come true.

What do you enjoy most about your work?
I love taking a director's concept of the characters from the script, hopefully adding something to it, then working it out with the actors. Enabling them in turn to embody the characters. With luck in the right direction it all comes alive on the screen.

And least?
Paperwork, including budget number crunching and politics.

What advice would you give to people trying to get into this area of work now?
It is difficult not to sound trite, but explore the craft, when working with people you admire learn everything you possibly can from them. Watch and learn all the time. Notice all types of make-up in life and on films, try to work out how it is done, replicate it on a chum, see if it works. If not then try to work it out.

When speaking to someone you wish to train with, know their work and the films they have worked on. Be engaged with filmmaking so you have at the very least an appreciation of other departments' work on a set. No one enjoys working with someone who has tunnel vision. Filmmaking is a group activity so selfishness in any department is detrimental to the film as a whole.

Make certain you want to do this work, rather than liking the idea of it. And lastly be determined.

Working on set

In film or motion pictures the words 'stage' and 'set' denote the area of work where shooting is going on. The make-up/hair artist should always ask at the start of filming whether the cameraman and director want the make-up personnel to step in between each shot to retouch make-up and hair or wait until they are called. When called, the assistant director will either ask for 'make-up' or 'checks' or 'final checks'. If a film star demands constant attention, the make-up artist and hair stylist should stand behind the camera, but not so close as to crowd the camera crew.

It is always important to work within the pattern of the director and cameraman's framework which will manifest itself on the first day's shoot. To save time when doing quick changes, a make-up place is often set up in a corner with a table and chair. Since the cameraman and director are concerned with the overall look, they will not notice if there are mistakes made concerning the make-up and hair until watching the film on screen. The fine detail is the responsibility of the make-up artist, whether powdering shiny faces, resticking the lace on a beard or prosthetic piece or applying fresh lipstick when needed. Time is always allowed for essential work such as applying blood in a fight scene, or tears and sweat at the appropriate moment.

What is the future?

The biggest industry shift involves the use of digital cameras. Photographers can send their pictures instantly across the world with a laptop and satellite phone. Films are already in production using digital cameras, such as George Lucas's *Star Wars, Attack of the Clones*. The end result is as good as 35mm film and the movie screens which already use digital projection show that the appearance is sharper and clearer than regular film. This is good news for future film-makers as the equipment is lighter and less expensive, which makes it easier for anyone to make a film, without costly film processing methods. It is also good news for TV and film technicians, particularly make-up artists. More than ever the make-up artist's work will need to be of the highest quality. There will be a demand for skilled make-up artists who can give the director what he wants with flair and speed.

Computers can create amazing effects, but will never replace actors or the make-up artists who transform or enhance their faces with make-up. In good and bad times people will wish to be entertained by drama, comedy and musicals. Films will always be made to satisfy that demand. Technology will help to deliver it.

Historical make-up and hair

7

Introduction

Researching the period for a production is one of the most interesting parts of a make-up artist's job. The history of the times that people lived in, what they wore, how they dressed their hair, what make-up they used and so on are continually fascinating. How authentic the final made-up look will be depends on the requirements of the production you are working on. Sometimes the style will be softened to suit current fashion, at others it will be accurate to the last detail.

In planning the make-up, pay attention to the character and age of the person whose role the actor is playing, as well as to the make-up used in the period. The notes given below are simply guidelines; you will need to adapt them to suit the look you wish to achieve.

Research

Period or historical make-up is closely tied to character work, but also linked to fashion as the overall look at a given time was based on the current fashion. Today's fashion will be tomorrow's period or historical make-up. The best way of researching is to study *old magazines* and *photographs*, to watch *old films* and to visit *museums* and *art galleries*.

Prehistoric people

The Natural History Museum in London provides evidence of prehistoric people, both in reconstructions and in pictures and books on anthropology. Another source of information is the cave drawings. They provide visual information and are the earliest known works of art by human beings.

The earliest records of Neanderthal man show a narrow receding forehead, with a broad flat nose and a heavy powerful jaw. The neck was heavy and the eye structure projected forward. People at this time were also very hairy. To achieve this look it would be necessary to use prosthetic appliances such as forehead pieces and dentures to project the jaw.

The Egyptians

The Egyptian civilisation, founded around 31 000BC, left a great deal of useful material in records of their culture. It is known that Egyptians shaved their heads and wore wigs made of hair from animals, humans and vegetable fibres. They wore plenty of make-up and were probably the first people to use black kohl, which is still worn today. Vegetable dyes, red clay and white lead were all used to adorn the faces of both sexes. The hair colour was usually black, but the wigs were sometimes dyed in bright shades of green, blue and red and the eyeshadow often matched the wig.

The eye make-up has become well known through archaeological evidence following the uncovering of buried tombs. The famous black lines drawn around the eyes from the inner corner and extended outward in a straight line 3 cm beyond the outer corner is the classic 'Cleopatra' style. The eyelashes and eyebrows were blackened and the brows extended. The cheeks and lips were reddened with carmine and the natural light-brown skin tone was often whitened with lead and oil foundations.

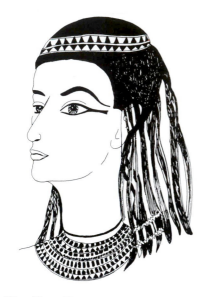

The Egyptians

The Greeks

The Greek civilisation around 350BC offered the ideal of the perfect face, still accepted today. A painted marble head, dating from 350BC and found in a Greek temple, depicts a fashionable lady of those days. The eyebrows are painted black, the upper eyelids are reddish-brown and dark green is used to emphasise the eye sockets. The same green is used as a strong eyeline on the lids close to the upper lashes and extended at the outer corners. The lips and cheeks are rouged a brownish-red colour.

The women had long hair and dressed it in elaborate styles, incorporating ringlets. Combs and jewels were used to decorate the hairstyle. The men did not wear wigs. Soldiers were clean-shaven and had their hair cut short and curled; many statues still exist which show the curled hair brushed forward. Some men dyed their hair blond or red and many of the elders had beards and moustaches.

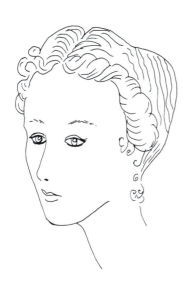

The Greeks

The Romans

A statue of a Roman beauty dating from the first century AD shows clearly her heavily darkened eyebrows. Most of the information about the use of make-up in those days comes from the writings of churchmen who objected to it during the early Christian period. In the fourth century St Ambrose called women 'harlots' for painting their faces. Because of the complaints of the Christian fathers we know that for three or four centuries after the birth of Christ many women were whitening their faces, necks and breasts, blackening their eyebrows and dyeing their hair. We know also that the lips and cheeks were reddened with magenta rouge. The fashionable colours for hair were blonde and red.

Pictorial evidence shows that the average Roman man had short hair and was clean shaven. The older men, intellectuals and philosophers had long hair and flowing beards.

The Middle Ages

The Middle Ages span the period 400–1500AD.

Mediaeval women used white lead to achieve a pale complexion, as the fashion for pale skins and red lips continued throughout Europe. A fourteenth-century sculpted Madonna from Spain shows plucked painted eyebrows, rouged lips and cheeks and black-lined eyes.

Many Dutch and French paintings dating from 1447–75 show plucked eyebrows and high, shaved foreheads. During the fourteenth and fifteenth centuries the women wore headdresses and removed any hair growing below the hairline. When not wearing a headdress the hair was long and dressed close to the head. The fashionable colours for hair were blonde and black, but not red.

Mediaeval men had long hair with flowing beards. By 1509, when Henry VII of England died, men's hair was worn shorter, with the facial hair trimmed. Hair had become less elaborate than earlier in the century.

Case Profile
Liz Michie, TV and film hairdresser

How did you get into the industry?

Thirty years ago I took a three-year City and Guilds course in hairdressing and wig making. This was the best grounding I could have had in my career. I worked in a hair salon for two years, then was lucky enough to pass an interview and complete a three-month training contract at the BBC. I spent three years there, before moving to Australia. I freelanced there for ten years, in film and TV, then returned to specialise in hair.

Who or what has been your most significant project?

One of the most significant projects was a four-hour American production called *The Mists Of Avalon* for TNT, filmed in Prague. Set in medieval times, it involved many wigs. I used many different techniques including sticking in weft extensions and lengthened a fairly short Merlin wig using pipe lagging, which worked very well.

What made it really special was all of the actors letting us do whatever we needed with no fuss. Top of the list was Joan Allen. I looked after her wig, which was made by Terry Jarvis. It included wefts, which I made into a ladder to extend the wig length. I also made some of the weft into small coils and plaits, which I used to decorate the wig.

What do you enjoy most about your work?

Every job is a brand new experience with a whole new set of crew and cast. I enjoy doing period work using wigs, probably because a wig can really change an actors' appearance.

And least?

Because of the long hours worked there is no time for a social life, and sometimes you can be working away on location for long periods of time. Your social life and work become intertwined and suddenly at the end of a contract you are without all the friends you have made. Having said all that I still consider myself privileged to be working in the film and TV industry.

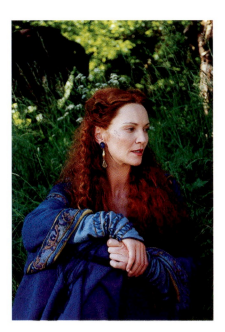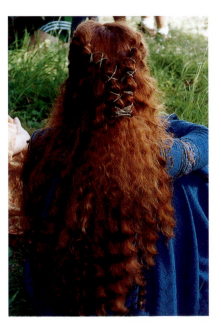

Make-up on Joan Allen by Liz Michie on *The Mists of Avalon*, TNT TV (US)

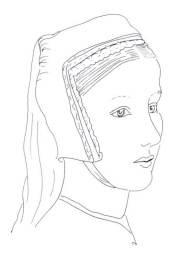

The sixteenth century

The sixteenth century

The Renaissance is the name given to that period which denoted the revival of arts, literature and science in Europe, bringing in a new style of architecture and decoration to succeed the Gothic.

Queen Elizabeth I (reigned 1558–1603) had red hair, which became fashionable. She also favoured heavy cosmetics. According to Ben Jonson and other writers of the day, the older she became, the heavier her application of cosmetics. During her reign the influence of the Renaissance first made itself felt in England. The dress, speech and manners of Italy became fashionable amongst her subjects.

Again, a white skin was desirable and white lead was still being used. People did not use natural plant extracts to obtain their colours for reddening the cheeks and lips, as in earlier centuries. Since this was the new scientific age, many artists' pigments were used for face-painting techniques and some of these were poisonous.

The seventeenth century

The French and English make-up and hairstyles became very similar when Charles I of England (reigned 1625–49) married Henrietta, the sister of Louis XIII of France (reigned 1610–43). It is important to remember that face painting has mainly been confined to sophisticated society in larger cities. Country people used little or no powder and paint and led healthier lives.

As the fashionable ladies of the English and French courts used more make-up, they started putting patches on their faces. The patches were in stars, half-moons and round shapes, cut out of black taffeta, Spanish leather or gummed paper. Such patches became useful for covering scars or skin afflictions and, according to reports of the day, gradually became excessive as women used more and more patches at a time. Famous portraits dating between 1670 and 1685 show that the fashionable look was a wide fleshy face with a double chin, prominent eyes, full red lips, dark eyebrows and dark hair.

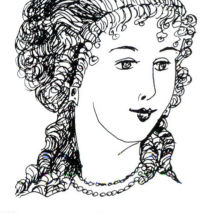

The seventeenth century

The Cavalier men wore their hair shoulder-length and curled. Their moustaches were curled, trimmed and pomaded or waxed. Beards became shorter and neater.

Puritan men cut their hair short and round and wore no facial hair. For this reason they were called Roundheads.

Louis XII started the fashion of wigs for men in France and Charles II of England popularised black wigs. The men were also using make-up. Judge Jeffreys, Lord Chancellor of England in 1678, was notorious for his extravagant use of make-up.

In Asia and Africa the make-up was entirely different from that used in Europe. From writers of the early seventeenth century (1603–25), we hear that many Moorish women were observed with tattoos on their faces and their bodies were coloured with henna.

The eighteenth century

The ladies at court continued to use heavy make-up, whitening their faces with lead paint and applying rouge heavily. They also powdered their shoulders and accentuated veins on the bosom with blue. By now there was publicity about the danger of using white lead paint and it was known that this eventually killed people. The fashion of using it still continued in England, however, and even more excessively in France, from where most of the cosmetics came.

The gentlemen also wore face paint and rouged their cheeks heavily. The fashion of powdering the hair or wig was very popular. White powder or flour was used by the nobility and soldiers. Moustaches and beards were out of fashion. The hair was still worn in a pigtail

The eighteenth century

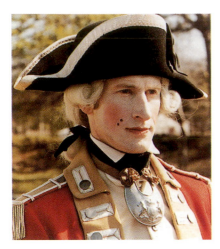

An English officer from the film *Revolution*

(or queue), using either the natural hair or a wig. Military men did not have facial hair at this time. By 1768 the men at court were blackening their eyebrows and reddening their lips.

Women's eyebrows were plucked thin, pencilled high and curved. Rouge was placed in a round or triangular shape. The lips were painted in a rounded shape with a 'bee-sting' effect.

The voluptuous look of the mid-seventeenth century had changed to the ideal of painted porcelain. By the middle of the century (1737–70) rouge was being placed in a round shape lower on the cheeks, in a bright pink colour. The lips were small and rosebud shaped, with paler eyebrows than previously.

Patches were still worn. During Queen Anne's reign (1702–14), patches became a political symbol, with Tories wearing their patches on the left side of the face and Whig supporters on the right. The wigs became larger and more fantastic until a tax on hair powdering was introduced in 1795. The excesses of this period came to an end with the French Revolution.

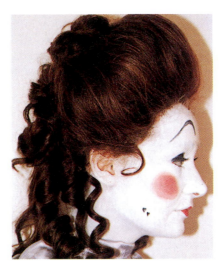

Eighteenth-century make-up Theatrical version

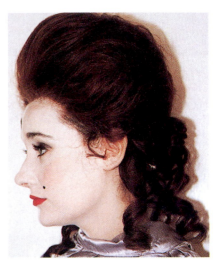

Film version

The nineteenth century

After the French Revolution, anything associated with the aristocracy went out of fashion. Wigs and long hair were out and most men had short hair. They began to grow sideburns and moustaches instead and by the middle of the century beards had also come into fashion. Wigs were retained only for the courts for official legal occasions.

Women wore cosmetics very discreetly. When Queen Victoria (reigned 1837–1901) came to the British throne there was a complete reaction against the use of any paint on the face. Women continued to use cosmetics, but since this was now considered vulgar they had to use even more discretion. Many cosmetics were home-made. Officially, powder creams and lotions were all that was used. Only stage actors and courtesans openly applied paints.

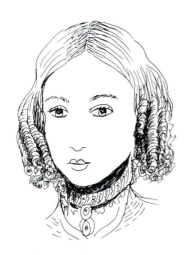

The nineteenth century

Meanwhile the men cultivated large handlebar moustaches with carefully curled ends. The women had long hair worn up in rolls and curls.

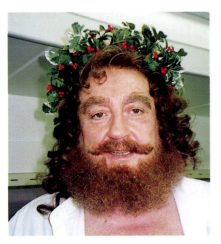

Step 1

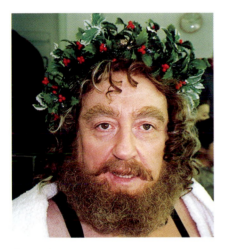

Step 2

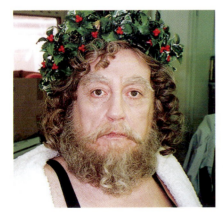

Step 3

Make-up, hair and instruction Tricia Cameron. Make-up and hair supervisor Norma Webb. Actor Desmond Barrit as the Ghost of Chistmas Present in *A Christmas Carol* for Hallmark

Step-by-step period hair and make-up

Brief

My brief was that the Ghost of Christmas Present was to age as Christmas Day passed into Christmas Night. I did it in five stages.

1 Desmond was wearing a wig, beard, moustache and eyebrows. The beard, wig and moustache were tightly dressed and the moustache was turned upwards. The base make-up was very healthy with red cheeks, and I highlighted any shadows to make him look as young as possible.

2 As money was at a premium, we used the same wig, to which I added some grey streaks, greyed the beard and moustache, made the beard narrower to bring the face in, the moustache was turned down a little and combed over the top lip. Rouge was removed from the cheeks.

3 A new wig was used which had a lot more grey in it, also a new beard, moustache and eyebrows, I started to reshape the beard to make the face longer and to make it more drawn, I added a greyer piece to the centre.

I changed the base to a paler one, still keeping it natural.

4 Still keeping the grey centrepiece in the beard I had added at stage three, the new beard was now much finer. I set it lower on the cheek area to make the face look longer and took a lot of the curl out of it so that it did not look as healthy as the ones before.

The base was now made even paler and I started to work on the shadowing around the eyes, nose and took the colour out of the lips.

5 Same wig, but redressed to make everything pull down, moustache brought down at the sides and centrepiece of beard taken off to make it seem thinner, grease put into the wig to make it look lank, hair taken off the forehead to make the head look longer. The beard was set even further back, and down on the chin.

The make-up was added too, with lots of shading, to make him look tired and worn out.

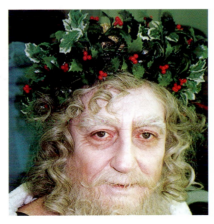

Step 4

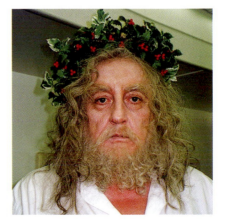

Step 5

Case Profile
Tricia Cameron, Hair and make-up designer and wig maker

How did you get into the industry?

I trained at the London College of Fashion, then became an assistant to the hair and make-up department at the Royal Opera House. From there I went to the Royal Shakespeare Company – until I was old enough to apply to the BBC. I have now been in the industry for thirty-three years.

What or who has been your most significant project?

This is a difficult one. I took over the hair department at Madame Tussaud's when I was just 20 years old. I was manager of the hair and make-up department at Glyndebourne Opera House at 26, working with designers such as Erte, David Hockney and Sir Hugh Casson. But, with my first film I reached the goal I had set myself.

What do you enjoy about your work?

Each new project is a challenge in one way or another. I never stop learning, which I find very exciting, and I never know what culture, era, or life I am going to dip into with the next job. I think I am extremely lucky to be in such a creative job and never knowing where or with whom I will be next.

What advice would you give to people trying to get into this area of work now?

They should learn everything they can, from anyone who is prepared to give them the time. Help out in whatever way you can and with good grace. You must love what you do as you will be asked to work long and hard. Be flexible – there is more than one right way for doing something. You must be able to work in a team, under supervision and to like people. Be patient, and if you want it that badly you will make it.

The twentieth century

Make-up was now being used to enhance rather than to overpaint the face. By 1913 light skin, dark eyebrows and full rosebud-shaped lips were the fashion. The hairstyles for women were still long and elaborately dressed on top of the head during the first decade. A style called the 'pompadour' was very fashionable.

The 1920s

In the 1920s a short haircut called the 'bob' became the vogue and the make-up that went with it created a new look. By 1925 the fashion was for a wistful look with soft, smudged eye make-up. The lips were painted red in a 'Cupid's bow' shape and the eyebrows were plucked, then redrawn in a thin arch sloping downwards at the ends. This gave a sad, wistful expression to the face. The skin was still pale and powdered to avoid shine.

From the late 1920s make-up was prepared using safe ingredients for the first time. Men were shaving off their facial hair at the beginning of the decade and any moustaches worn were always neatly clipped. The hairstyles were short, neat and plastered down to the head, usually in a side parting.

1920s Make-up

1   Using a fair coloured pancake make-up, cover the entire face (including the lips). Solidify the look with a translucent powder.

2   Block out the eyebrows using a bar of wet soap completely covering the entire eyebrow area.

3   Using camouflage make-up, colour over the soap with skin tones completely hiding the white. Create a thin eyebrow using a black eyeliner pencil.

4   Use a deep black eyeshadow over the entire crease of the eye. Add black eyeliner and black mascara.

5   Place a deep red on the lips creating the cupid bow 1920s look. Use camouflage to block out the natural lip shape remaining.

6   Style hair using minimal curls and maintaining short cropped style.

The process takes around $1\frac{1}{2}$ hours.

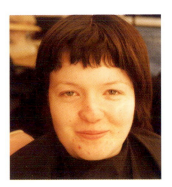

Before

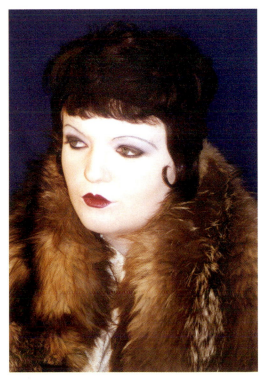

Make-up Artist
Shauna O'Toole.
Model Meineer Rees   After

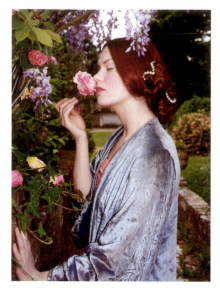

Make-up artist Shauna O'Toole.
Model Camilla Tew

J.W. Waterhouse painting recreation

1   Collect appropriate props including fake flowers, clothing, pearls, wig, pancake make-up.
2   Style the wig and weave the pearls into the twist braid.
3   Apply pale pancake make-up over the entire model (face and exposed body parts).
4   Use pink pancake make-up on the cheeks to create a very rosy and painted look.
5   Use a deeper mauve colour on the natural lip line.
6   Line the eyebrows with a deep brown.
7   Place the wig on the model and the appropriate clothes for the photo.

The process takes around 30 minutes.

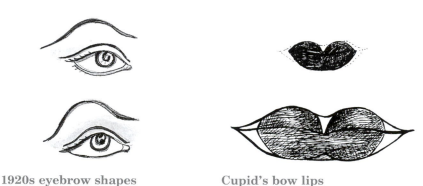

1920s eyebrow shapes   Cupid's bow lips

1930s eyebrow shape

The 1930s

During the 1930s the women started painting their lips in a more natural shape and making the mouth look wider rather than smaller. The foundations were natural coloured and still powdered heavily. Rouge or blusher was applied lower, under the cheekbones. Eyeshadow was blended from the eyelids up to the eyebrows, in subtle smoky blues and browns. Lipstick was still red. The eyebrows were not too heavily plucked.

The styles were set by Hollywood films. Hair was bleached blonde and waved tightly with irons. Nail varnish was used in both bright and dark colours.

The men had short neat hairstyles and moustaches of different shapes, but no beards.

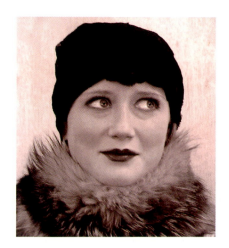

The early 1930s

The 1940s

In the 1940s, during the Second World War, less make-up was used in England, simply because it was unavailable. The one available item was lipstick, which was a symbol of the era. As well as red lipstick, the 1940s look relied on natural-looking eyebrows, brushed into shape and darkened.

Women's hair was usually worn long, with more natural-looking waves than in the previous two decades. In 1941 the film star Veronica Lake set a fashion with her long hair undulating in waves and falling across one side of her face.

Postiche hairpieces were used for styles requiring curls or chignons when dressing the hair. Wigs had been used for some time, but they were unobtrusively named 'transformations'.

Men had short hair still, but cultivated waves in it using a comb and water. They too were influenced by the film stars. In England men wore moustaches, but in America these were unusual, apart from the 'Clark Gable' shape which was sometimes seen.

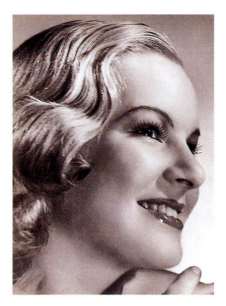

The early 1940s

Room for Two (1940)

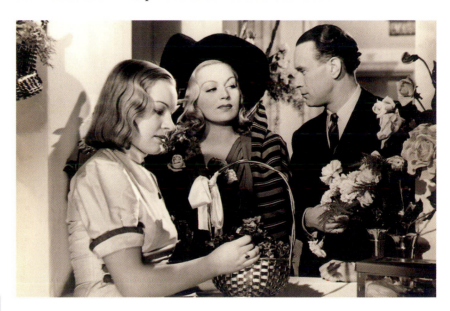

The 1950s

By the 1950s make-up had become more natural looking. The products were of a better quality and there was more choice in colours than ever before. The Hollywood musicals in glorious Technicolor seemed to bring a fashion in brighter skin tones. Suntans became fashionable as people were able to travel freely after the war. A fake tan for men, called 'Man Tan', was popular. Women had more choice in lipstick shades and corals, oranges and vivid pinks were much in demand. The eyes were not heavily made up. The look was an all-over one without particular emphasis on one feature.

In the mid-1950s the 'Mandarin' look arrived from Paris. The outer ends of the eyebrows were entirely plucked and redrawn in an

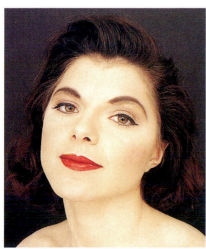

The 1950s

upward sweep. The eyelines were drawn upwards at the outer corners. The rest of the face had no colour, except the lips – overall an interesting effect.

The hairstyles became shorter, fuller and curlier. Blonde was still a popular colour in American films and the fashions were taken from current filmstars – Marilyn Monroe, Elizabeth Taylor and Doris Day. Audrey Hepburn set a fashion for a doe-eyed look, with heavy black eyelines.

Chignons and false hair were popular. Then in 1953 the Italian filmstars started a fashion called the 'Italian cut' – a short, shaggy-looking hairstyle. This was popular for a while and then gave way to the bouffant style: a thick pageboy style, puffed out at the sides and lacquered heavily to hold it in place.

The men had shaven faces and short hair at the back and sides, with long hair at the front worn in a tuft or wave, like Elvis Presley. Crew cuts were also popular. Less conservative men wore beards and moustaches.

The 1960s

The 1960s saw a decade of rebellion, in which the younger generation switched to a completely different appearance, with many different fashions, each more bizarre than the last.

For women eye make-up dominated the decade. In 1962 the Egyptian look was fashionable, with heavy black eyelines and strong eyebrows. In 1963 the lips seemed to disappear. No colour was added to them and attention was focused on the heavy eye make-up.

In 1965 the eyebrows were played down as well as the lips, so the eyes were the focal point, with heavy colouring and false eyelashes. This was a very theatrical look, with heavy shading in the eye sockets and pale colour or none on the eyelids. The lips were pale. Sometimes they were painted with frosted pink or any chalky-looking colour. Rouge or blusher was not used, but shading was added under the cheekbones to add emphasis to the face shape.

The 1960s

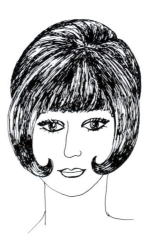
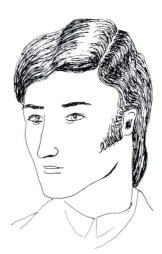

Men grew their hair long and sideburns, moustaches and beards were fashionable.

Women wore their hair in elaborate styles, hairpieces being used more generally to make their hair look larger and fuller. A style called the 'beehive' became popular and it became so large in size that it looked like a soldier's busby.

'Flower power' became fashionable, with young people 'dropping out' and rebelling against the work ethic. They were called 'hippies' and wore their hair very long and deliberately unkempt looking.

The 1970s

The 'flower power' movement lasted in England until 1975. Eye make-up was slightly softer than in the 1960s, with frosted eyeshadows and painted bottom lashes. A shiny doll-like look became fashionable, with glossy pastel colours painted on the lips, eyelids and cheekbones. The men still had long hair, though it was not popular in the workplace.

By 1975 an aggressively unglamorous look called 'punk' had swept away all traces of the 1960s. Heads were fully or partially shaved and safety pins worn through the nose. The look was deliberately hard and ugly. Tattoos started to become fashionable and girls had pale faces with no make-up or heavily painted eye make-up.

The 1970s

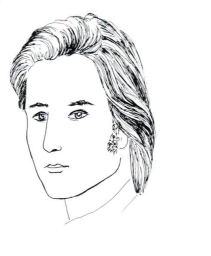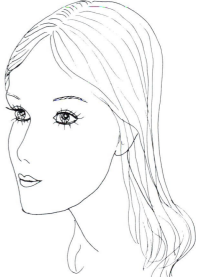

The 1980s

In the 1980s the punk look gave way to the 'Gothic' look. Faces were painted white once more with heavy, dark eye make-up and hair being gelled to make it stick up.

The rest of the population conformed to a different fashion. Hairstyles became 'big' for women, to match their expensive designer clothes with large shoulder pads. Waves of fashions sought to create past styles such as the 1940s. A unique style was the fashion for heavy ungroomed eyebrows for women, a look started by the film actress Brooke Shields who had naturally heavy eyebrows. The make-up became quite strong for women, with blusher being swept across the tops of the cheekbones. For a while, pink was used on the eyelids.

Men's hair became short again, with 1950s hairstyles in fashion. The 1980s were boom years and the young business people, called 'yuppies', tended to be materialistic, spending their money lavishly on clothes and grooming. However, the boom finished with the decade and the world plunged into recession.

The 1980s

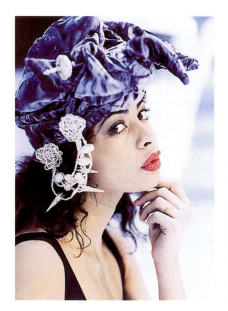

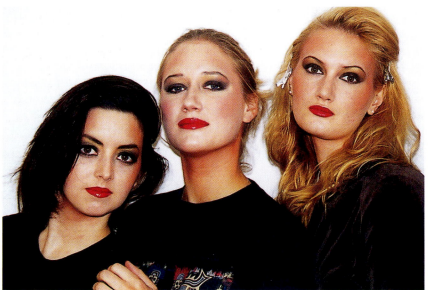

The 1990s

Nostalgia became popular, with fashion adopting looks from past decades, revamping and adopting them as its own. The models on the catwalks went swiftly through a 1960s revival at the beginning of the 1990s, bringing false eyelashes back into fashion. Eyebrows were shaved off for a while and a line pencilled in, but this did not catch on with the general public. The 'grunge' look with unmade-up faces and untidy hair became popular with young people.

There were also 1930s and 1950s revivals and hairstyles ranged from elegant upswept chignons to braided plaits and layered bobs reminiscent of past eras. One fashion unique to the first half of the 1990s (1990–4) was the fashion for large lips. Not only did the famous models overpaint their mouths to look as large as possible, but some had silicon injections to give a particularly swollen look to the upper lip.

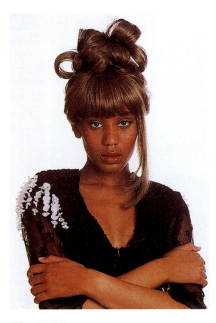

The 1990s

When choosing cosmetics, many people went back to ancient times when the pigments used were derived from plant extracts. The popularity of homeopathic medicine helped to promote a preference for natural-based products. On the whole, the fashion in make-up and hair was based on a natural look, achieved through a more skilful application of face paints than in the past.

Period hairstyles

As with period make-up, researching period hairstyles will involve visiting museums, art galleries and libraries, and looking at magazines, old photographs and so forth. Here are some simple examples, from the Egyptian period through to the twentieth century, which should serve as a useful guide.
(See also pages 134–47 for some background information on period hairstyles.)

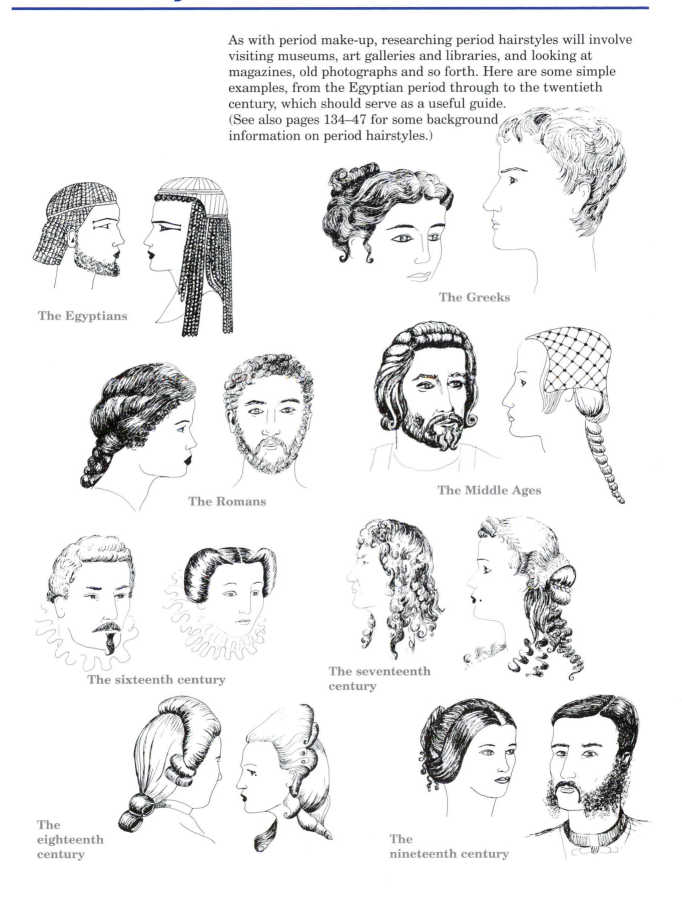

The Egyptians

The Greeks

The Romans

The Middle Ages

The sixteenth century

The seventeenth century

The eighteenth century

The nineteenth century

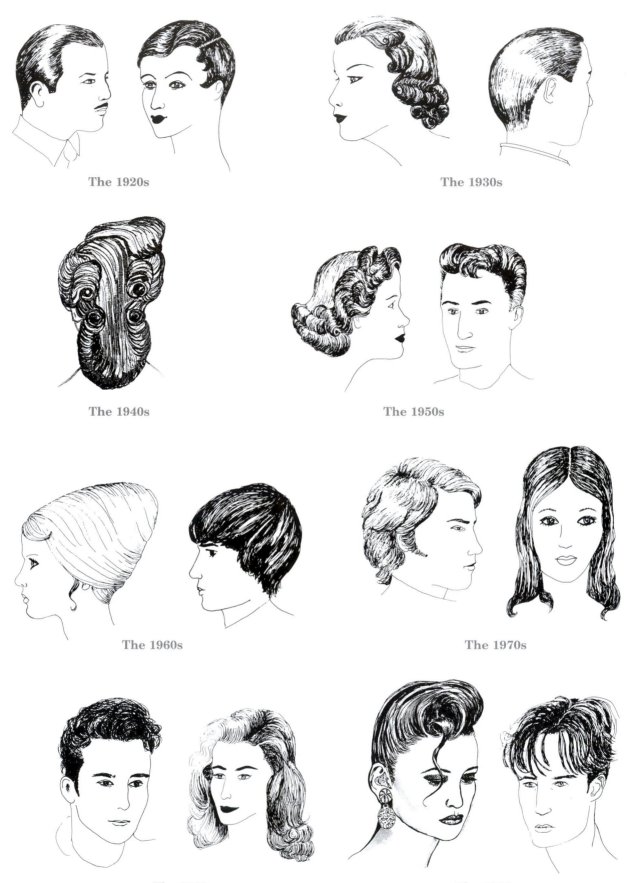

The 1920s

The 1930s

The 1940s

The 1950s

The 1960s

The 1970s

The 1980s

The 1990s

Adapting fashion make-up to period styles

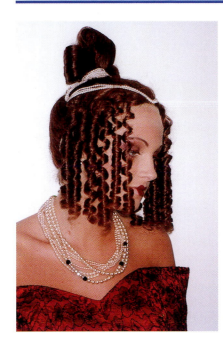

The period look adapted to modern fashion

Some faces adapt easily to period styles. You will often hear a make-up artist remark that a certain actress has a 'period face'. It is not always possible in period productions for TV and films to reproduce faithfully the 'correct' historical look. The effect may be distracting or considered too ugly relative to the current fashion. Often it is necessary instead to indicate the period by conveying the *feeling* of the look.

For example, in the Restoration period white head paint was used as a base. You could use a cream panstik for a heavy authentic look, but it might be necessary to use a thin, pale, liquid base so that the effect was not too theatrical. Pure white is often a problem for the lighting, making it necessary to use a beige or cream base instead. Similarly, if the period look includes plucked eyebrows but the current fashion is for natural, heavy brows, then the audience would not want the leading actress to look 'bizarre', even if her make-up were historically correct.

The Victorian period is easy: for this the actor should look as if she or he is not made-up at all, as make-up was not supposed to be worn. The facial hair on the men and the women's hairstyles are more important in conveying the historical look.

Actors must be comfortable in their roles. Remember, for example, that in the 1940s not every man had a moustache. On the other hand, if the actor is meant to be an RAF pilot, he will be more believable with a moustache since this was certainly fashionable at the time, especially amongst aircrew. Wherever possible, do try to get the period right.

 Activity – Two eighteenth-century looks

1 Apply an eighteenth century make-up to your model. Try to reproduce an authentic historical style, as you think it would have looked in those days (see notes below.)

2 Adapt today's fashion to an eighteenth-century look. This time, show how you would do it for a film today.

Notes: For the hair, use a white powdered wig with a combination of rolls and two curls. Add a piece on the top of the head to give greater height. If you do not have a wig, make one out of cottonwool to get the right effect, or spray a dark wig with white spray.

Take photographs of each make-up. Compare the results and discuss the differences.

Activity – Creating a dramatic look

From the 1920s to the present day, the dramatic effect of a pale face with defined eyebrows, blood-red lips and intense eyes has been ever-popular.

Use compressed eyeshadows, in matt dark shades of charcoal grey, dark aubergine, dark brown or black, along the eye sockets and beneath the bottom eyelashes, to give a sultry look.

Activity – Creating cupid's-bow lips

1 With the mouth slightly open, apply red lipstick: from the centre of the upper lip, in upward and outward curves to the apex and then down, with a round movement, towards the corners. Do not carry the lipstick to the extreme corners, as this would make the mouth look large and wide.

   Take care that the two curves are of equal size, or the lip will look one-sided. Keep the curves slightly separated, or the mouth will appear to pout.

2 For the lower lip, place the colour in the centre and then blend it to right and left. Leave as much unpainted space at the corners as in the upper lip.

Activity – Creating a 1970s 'flower power' look

1 Use soft translucent colours (pink, orange and peach) to create a soft-focus look.
2 Use pale blue frosted eyeshadow on the eyes.
3 Leave the eyebrows bare, or pencil in thin lines.
4 Paint Cupid's-bow lips in pale colours and accentuate with lip gloss.
5 Highlight eyebrow bones with pale colours (cream, beige or pale pink).

Hairdressing and wigmaking

8

Introduction

In feature film production it is customary to employ hairdressers to design and dress the actors' hair, but in television it is often the make-up artist who is required to do the *hairdressing*. For commercials and fashion photographic work make-up artists are usually expected to have both skills. In theatre, on the other hand, there are usually wig departments to meet these needs and actors will apply their own make-up. To be able to secure work in any area of the industry – film, TV, videos, commercials, fashion photography and pop promotions – the student make-up artist is therefore wise to learn as much as possible about hairdressing.

Often you will be working with the artiste's own hair. At other times you will be preparing added hair (*postiche*) as a wig or facial hairpiece. Colleges throughout the country offer courses in hairdressing, most leading to some kind of qualification. As well as acquiring the basic hairdressing skills of cutting, setting and dressing hair, the make-up student needs to learn special skills, such

Wigs dressed and ready to be attached to the head

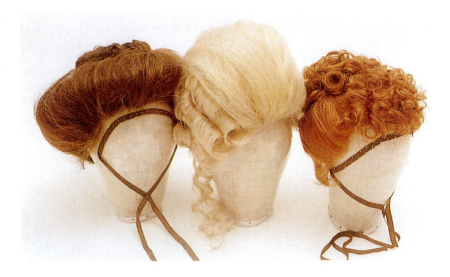

as how to adapt a modern hairstyle to resemble a historical style for a period film or TV production and how to *break down* hair so that it looks naturally untidy or dirty. You must learn:

- how to clean, block and dress a wig
- how to prepare the artiste's own hair for application of a wig or hairpiece
- how to fit and secure the wig or hairpiece
- how to dress out the wig or hairpiece on the artiste's head
- how to apply and remove temporary colouring for particular hair effects

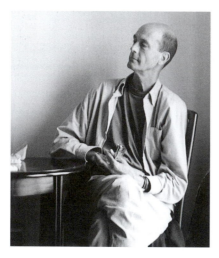

Ken Lintott

Case Profile
Ken Lintott, Make-up and hair designer

When and how did you start in the business?

I started as an outside supplier, making headdresses for the aborted 1960 *Cleopatra* film (for Wig Creations). This was after art school where I studied stage design and worked on many amateur and university productions.

Was there a turning point in your career?

Being trained at Wig Creations, progressing through wigmaking to wig design on theatre, film and TV productions: this led to setting up the make-up and wig departments of the Royal Shakespeare Companies at Stratford upon Avon and London, Aldwych, which was the turning point in my career. I later freelanced as wigmaker and make-up artist on films, opera, ballet and TV, as well as theatre, both at home and abroad.

What do you think are the important qualities for a make-up artist?

Patience, skill and expertise in all the techniques required, as well as adaptability, humour and enormous energy. Loyalty to your colleagues, along with punctuality and reliability.

How has your career changed your life?

It has enabled me to fulfil early artistic yearning, enabling me to contribute to the overall scope of productions and to work with some extraordinarily talented colleagues.

What have been your most satisfying jobs?

First, pioneering and developing early inventions for 'bald caps' and the like. Second, passing on skills to young people.

What advice would you give to people trying to get into this area of work now?

Learn hard and be prepared to work very hard.

Do you think the TV/film world is glamorous?

The 'glamour' of the TV/film/theatre world is completely illusory and has nothing to do with a day's (or night's) work.

What do you consider the best and worst aspects of being a make-up artist?

The best aspect is the satisfaction of a job well done, on time and part of an overall excellence in all departments. The worst is, without doubt, surviving extreme temperatures, on location at night, especially around 3.30 am.

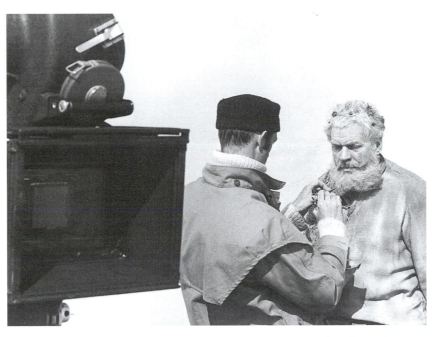

Ken Lintott preparing Paul Scofield for a take in *King Lear*, 1968. Paul's beard is overlaid with loose hair and brambles for when Lear is 'mad'

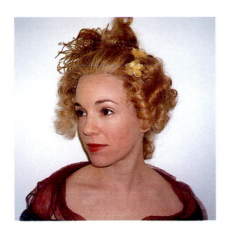

Period hairstyle

The hairstyle

Just as lighting and shading with make-up can dramatically change the shape of the face, so the hairstyle can alter the shape of the head, accentuating a strong feature or disguising a weak one. A good hairstyle, in conjunction with the make-up, suggests the period, the character and the age. Equally, however, the effect of a skilful make-up can be ruined if the hairstyle is unsuitable for the character.

 Activity – Studying the effects of hairstyles

On a piece of paper, draw a series of copies of the same head shape. Now sketch in the hair in various styles and look at the changes the different styles make to the way the head looks.

As in other aspects of make-up, *continuity* is important. It sometimes seems in film and television work that if a lock of hair is placed differently in one shot from the next, everyone notices. Because of the natural movement of hair, its position must be monitored closely during filming.

Postiche

The term postiche is French in origin and includes all added hairpieces – wigs, transformations, pincurls, switches, fringes, falls, backpieces, toupees, fronts and every other kind of article made

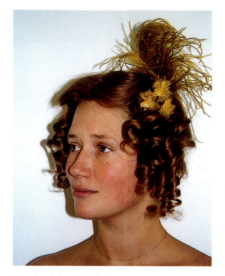

Period hairstyle

with hair. Years ago, each hairdressing salon had its own workroom in which postiche was made to order. In this workroom the student hairdressers first handled hair and learnt to appreciate its texture. They studied the way hair falls into waves and curls and learnt to manipulate it with ease. Gradually they acquired a feel for the craft, developing knowledge and skill in the handling of growing hair and making of postiche. When short hair became widespread, this form of craftsmanship dwindled. Few salons now have practical understanding of postiche work and hairpieces have to be ordered from specialists. The demand continues in film, television and theatre work, of course. No doubt the circle of fashion will eventually turn and postiche will again be required by the public.

The make-up artist's responsibilities

For a large-scale production there may be as many as 20 wigs, plus numerous falls, headpieces and added facial hairpieces. If a character in the production ages extensively, the same actor may need several different wigs from youth through to old age. If stunt doubles are being used, duplicate wigs may be needed.

The make-up artist (or hair designer) must first specify what is required, providing drawings, diagrams, reference photographs, written notes and perhaps verbal descriptions. Each wig must include a mixture of shades of the chosen colour, otherwise it will look dull and unconvincing. With the right mixture of colours in the wig or facial hair, a character can be made to look stronger or more vibrant. Remember too that a man's hair, eyebrows, beard and moustache may not all be of the same colour.

Wigs blocked and dressed

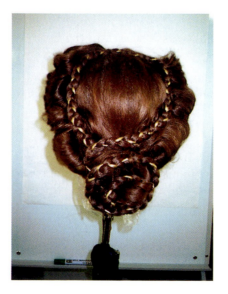

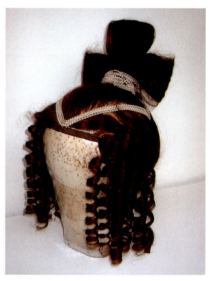

Although some postiche can be hired, much will have to be bought. Occasionally it will be possible to *refront* an existing wig to ensure correct fit for re-use. Before hiring, several companies must be contacted and the one selected that offers the best price and workmanship. Facial hair cannot be hired and has only a short lifespan. Moustaches, beards, sideburns and eyebrows are made to order in any size, shape or colour. For a long TV series purchase will prove cheaper than repeating hiring.

The make-up artist must oversee the wigmaking process and ensure that all the postiche items required are delivered on time, before shooting begins. The principal actors will need several fittings, whether the wig is being made specially or altered to fit them. During production, the wigs must be cleaned and dressed at the end of each day, ready for use on the next.

A wig with too much hair knotted into it will look false. If the hairlace at the edges is too thick or too white, this will show on camera. To understand such characteristics and to be able to judge what constitutes a good wig, you need to have learnt about the wigmaking process.

Equipment for making postiche

Types of hair used in postiche work

Human hair

Human hair tends to be used solely for wigs and hairpieces. The most expensive is eyebrow hair, particularly if it is blond, red or grey. The main countries supplying human hair for wigs are Italy and Spain. Asian hair is more common and therefore less expensive; as it is usually dark, Asian hair needs to be lightened.

Cleaning and dyeing processes weaken the hair and make it porous. Because the hair no longer has its natural supply of oil, it does not behave as it would on the head, either in its movement or in the way it holds any curl.

When handling a swatch of human hair, it is important to keep the *root* ends of the hair (the clubbed ends) lying in the same direction.

Yak hair

Yak hair is used for facial hairpieces – beards, eyebrows, sideburns and moustaches – and for chest wigs and the like. The softer hair is from the belly of the yak, the coarser hair from the tail. Yak hair is dyed by the hair merchant to match the required colour.

If the hair needs to be curled, it can be permed on rods after the piece has been knotted. Alternatively, it can be pre-curled on rods in a pressure cooker and dried in an oven before knotting. These processes usually result in a colour change, so the final facial hairpieces may not exactly match the hair sample. Using pre-curled hair usually gives a better finish to the moustache, but curled hair is also more difficult to knot.

Wool crepe hair

Wool crepe hair is the cheapest type of hair, and comes braided over two strands of cord which are removed before using the hair. Wool crepe hair does not have long hairs but consists of many shorter hairs, held together by overlapping.

Colours

Wool crepe hair comes in many colours, with shades of blond, brown, black, grey, red and white. These look natural when mixed. Unusual colours also are available, such as bright green or yellow. White braids can be dyed any colour using normal wool dyes, or sprayed with hair-colouring materials.

Uses

In the larger theatres and auditoriums and occasionally in TV and film for extras in the background, wool crepe hair is mainly used for facial hair. It is also used in hairstyles as padding, to give extra bulk to the existing hair, whether natural or in a wig.

Preparation

1 Cut a piece of braided wool crepe hair, about 300 mm long.
2 Remove the two cords.
3 Straighten the hair by dipping it in hot water.
4 Wrap it carefully in a towel, to absorb excess water.
5 Dry the hair by winding it round the back of a chair and leaving it overnight or, to dry the hair more quickly, use a hand-held dryer.
6 When completely dry, cut the hair into shorter lengths (about 150 mm).
7 Each length should be teased apart carefully and divided into smaller widths (about 25 mm across).
8 Hold a small bunch of hair in the middle and use a wide-toothed metal comb on the ends of the hair.
9 Using sharp scissors, cut off the straggly ends to make the strands even in length.
10 Repeat the combing and cutting with each bunch and lay them carefully on tissue paper or facial tissues. Fold over the tissues to store the hair for future use.

Mixing shades

First prepare the different shades or colours of wool crepe hair as above. Then combine them as follows:

1   Place one small mat of prepared hair on top of another.

2 Pull the ends to tug the hair apart into two sections.

3 Continue mixing the colours by laying one colour on top of another and pulling the hair apart, until the desired effect is achieved.

Real crepe hair

Real crepe hair is braided together in the same way as wool crepe hair, but consists of human or animal hair. When the cords have been removed the skeins are usually 150 mm or 200 mm in length.

The hair can be straightened by using a steam iron. It is then prepared with a **hackle** in the same way as other real hair. A hackle is a giant comb used to disentangle hair and for mixing hair for colour matching.

Angora goat hair

Angora goat hair is very soft and fine and therefore suitable for specialised wigs such as period powder wigs, or for soft-looking beards such as Father Christmas beards. It is usually blended with yak hair for beards and added as necessary to other hair to provide softness.

Horsehair

Horsehair is stiff and straight. It is used for barristers' and judges' wigs. It is also useful for adding whiskers to an animal make-up.

Artificial hair

Wigs and hairpieces can be obtained in artificially created *plastic hairs*. These are available in department stores and specialist shops. Although much less expensive than real hair (either animal or human), artificial hair is more difficult to dress. However, it is very tough and long lasting, so many rented wigs for period work are made of artificial hair. They are suitable for theatre productions but not used much in TV or film work as they are less natural looking than real-hair work.

On low-budget productions, artificial hair wigs are very useful and do not require much maintenance. They can be cleaned by gently immersing in lukewarm water mixed with a mild wig cleanser or fabric softener. They should be rinsed in cold water several times and then left to drip-dry naturally.

Lace

The types of **hair lace** or *gauze* range from thick theatre lace, used mainly in large theatres, to very fine laces, used by film and TV productions and where a theatre production is to be staged in a small space such as a studio. Although the thicker, coarser types of laces last longer, they tend to allow less movement of the face and can therefore be less comfortable for the actor.

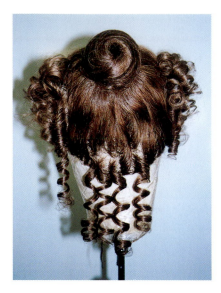

A period wig

Film and TV lace come in two thicknesses, 30 denier and 20 denier (which is finer). It requires greater skill and care to knot facial pieces on 20 denier lace, as this is prone to tearing. Never use a piece of lace with a snag or fault in it as this will inevitably become a large hole during the knotting process. Thick lace will loosen a little once it has been cleaned several times.

The shades of lace vary slightly, from off-white to darker tones. Before knotting, lace can be stained somewhat darker using a weak solution of tea. If the facial piece is required for black skin, *potassium permanganate solution* can be used to dye the lace dark brown.

Knotting hooks

Knotting hooks come in a range of sizes. For knotting the bulk of a wig you would use a hook capable of picking up six or seven hairs at a time. For the front hairline of a wig you would use a finer hook, as here you want to pick up only one hair at a time. Facial hair likewise needs a fine hook.

The *angle* of the hook can be altered to suit the individual. *Hook holders* are made either of plastic or of brass; the latter is heavier. These too come in differing lengths. A fairly large hook is used in whipping together with nylon thread the pleats on wig foundations and beards. Such hooks are sometimes called *whipping hooks*.

Making a wig

A wig can change a person's appearance almost beyond recognition. The height of the forehead can be increased and the width extended, for example, and an actor with a bald head can be transformed with a convincing head of hair, provided that it is a good wig and properly suited to the character. Wigs are made according to two main principles:

- those which can be blended to tone into the general make-up, which use a gauze or net front, the *hair lace*
- those which provide a full head of hair without the need to blend the make-up – these have no hair-lace fronts and are known as *hard-front wigs*.

The wigs fronted with hair lace are used in TV and film make-up as they are more natural looking in camera close-ups. Hair-lace wigs are very expensive. They also demand greater skill and care in fitting than the hard-fronted wigs.

The less expensive, hard-fronted wigs are used in the theatre and are easier to put on, requiring no extra attention with the make-up as the edge of the wig provides the dividing line at the hairline.

The fitting of a wig must be as perfect as possible, so meticulous care should be taken in measuring the actor or in selecting from stock. Once the make-up artist has begun making up the actor on a shoot, there is no time to rectify any errors in the fit of the wig.

Taking measurements for a wig

WIG SPECIALITIES LTD.
173 SEYMOUR PLACE · LONDON · W.1

NAME: ....

CHARACTER: ....

DATE: ....

MEASUREMENTS TAKEN BY: ....

WIG MEASUREMENTS

1.	CIRCUMFERENCE AROUND HEAD	☐ ins.
2.	FRONT TO BACK	☐ ins.
3.	TEMPLE TO TEMPLE AROUND BACK OF HEAD	☐ ins.
4.	EAR TO EAR OVER CROWN	☐ ins.
5.	NAPE OF NECK	☐ ins.
6.	TOP OF EAR TO NAPE OF NECK	☐ ins.
7.	EAR TO EAR OVER FOREHEAD	☐ ins.
8.	TEMPLE TO TEMPLE ACROSS FACE	☐ ins.

PARTING ☐ RIGHT ☐ LEFT ☐ CENTRE ☐ NONE

TOUPEE MEASUREMENTS

1.	LENGTH	☐ ins.
2.	TEMPLE	☐ ins.
3.	CROWN	☐ ins.
4.	BACK	☐ ins.

PARTING ☐ RIGHT ☐ LEFT ☐ CENTRE ☐ NONE

ARTICLE ....

PERIOD OR TYPE OF WIG ....

WEIGHT OF HAIRPIECE ☐ THICK ☐ THIN ☐ SPARSE

HAIR LENGTH ☐ ins.

COLOUR ....

DRESSING ☐ CURLY ☐ WAVY ☐ STRAIGHT

DIRECTION OF COMBING ....

REMARKS ....

....

....

....

....

NOTE – WHEREVER POSSIBLE SUPPLY SKETCH OF THE STILLS OF THE ARTIST WITH THIS FORM.

Preparation

Although as a make-up artist you will not have to make wigs yourself, it is useful to understand the wigmaking process. This will help you when commissioning or hiring wigs. The process of making a good-quality wig uses a special knotting hook to knot small bunches of real hair onto a *foundation* base of gauze or hair lace. This process is similar to the way in which carpets or rugs are made and many actors refer to their toupee or wig as their 'rug'.

The foundation on which the hair is knotted is fixed to a wooden **block** with small nails called *block points*. The block is held in position by means of a clamp attached to the edge of a table or workbench. The loose hair used for knotting is held in place using a **drawing mat** or *card*.

Equipment and materials

- clingfilm
- clear adhesive tape
- pencil (soft)

Making a pattern

The head measurements must be taken in order to make a *pattern* of the head on which the foundation can be based. As an example look at the chart used by a wig company to specify the details required in order to make a wig or toupee. Usually the actor is taken by the make-up artist to the wig company for a consultation and fitting. If this is impossible, the chart is made and sent to the wig company.

Traditionally the pattern was made by transferring the measurements of the head to a piece of paper, which was then cut and shaped. Nowadays wigmakers use clingfilm, a method which is easier and more accurate. When the measurements and pattern are ready, they are sent to the wigmaker.

Making a pattern for a wig

1 Prepare the head by brushing the hair back from the face and as close to the head as possible.

2 Wrap clingfilm tightly around the head, towards the back. A single piece should be big enough to wrap the front of the head and fasten at the back. If there is a gap on top of the head, fill this in with another piece of clingfilm.

3 Now secure this with clear adhesive tape. First apply the tape over the top of the head from ear to ear, making sure it is not too tight. Next take adhesive tape from the front to the back. Then apply tape along the entire circumference. Cover the whole head in this way until the pattern feels rigid, like a stiff cap.

4 Now draw in the existing hairline with a soft pencil, from the front, around the ear and down to the nape of the neck. If the hair is fine at the hairline, draw fine lines. Cover the pencil line with adhesive tape to protect it.

5 Remove the pattern from the head by easing it off gently.

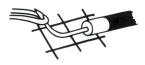

Single knotting –
A small quantity of hair is placed in drawing mats with the ends protruding. A few hairs at a time are drawn out and turned over to form a loop held in the left hand; this is dampened. The knotting hook is inserted under one mesh of the lace and one or several hairs are picked up from the loop in the left hand

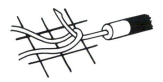

This loop is drawn under and through the hole in the lace

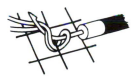

The hook is turned to catch the remaining ends of hair

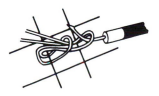

These ends are pulled carefully through the loop on the hook towards the right-hand side

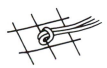

The completed knot is pulled tight so that it is as invisible as possible (dampening the hair at the outset helps this). Care should be taken to ensure that both ends of the hair are always pulled through

Making the foundation

The wigmaker cuts the pattern at the back and places it on the right-sized wooden block. The edges are then taped back together and the pattern is fixed with points. The wooden block used to make postiche should be approximately 15 mm larger than the circumference of the artiste's head. If the block is too small it should be padded. A cut is made and tissue paper pushed through; the cut is resealed with clear adhesive tape. Further cuts are made elsewhere as necessary. Only one cut is made at a time and never too near the hairline.

The foundation, mount or base is now made using net, gauze or silk. Springs, ribbons and fasteners provide extra support and fit. *Galloon*, a type of silk ribbon, is sewn around the outline of the pattern. The foundation net is sewn onto the galloon and this forms the shape of the wig base. For a more natural-looking frontal hairline, a galloonless edge is more suitable. This applies to wigs or hairpieces used in TV and film work. Once the wig foundation has been made to measure, it is ready for knotting.

Knotting

As a make-up artist you are not required to make wigs, but you do need to understand how they are made in order to recognise good workmanship. Knotting, however, does have practical applications. One such is knotting in extra hairs to soften and generally improve the appearance of a damaged or poorly knotted hairline.

Knotting is a delicate operation, requiring patience and good eyesight. It takes practice and time to become an expert knotter. To start with you should practise on odd pieces of foundation net, attached to a block with block points. It is best to use straight hair about 150 mm in length. Select a knotting needle to suit the size of the mesh of the net and firmly secure this into the wooden handle.

Types of knotting

There are many different types of knots. Those generally used in making a wig are described below.

Single knotting

In single knotting, individual knots of hair are added to the foundation net. This is the most common method of knotting when fine net is used. Different sizes of hooks can be used, depending on the amount of hair needed for each knot.

Double knotting

Double knots are tied to make the hair absolutely secure. The result is more unsightly as the knots are less easily concealed. **Double knotting** is used on the crown and large parts of the foundation, but single knotting is usually employed for the more visible parts of the wig.

Point knotting

Point knotting is single knotting the point ends of the hair. The root ends are cut away, allowing the hair to lift from the piece. This technique is useful for men's short-haired postiche, on the nape of a short-haired woman and on light fringes.

Underknotting

After the piece has been knotted, it is turned inside out on a malleable block. Single knotting is applied around the edge of the foundation, following the direction of the hair on the other side. Two or three rows of underknotting can be added. The wig is usually pressed when finished, using tissue paper or cloth to protect the hair.

Knotting a hairline on a film wig

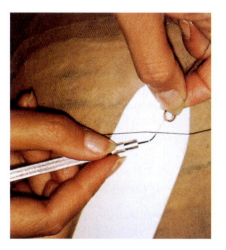

Hand knotting into the hairline: a white card has been inserted to make the very fine lace visible for working on

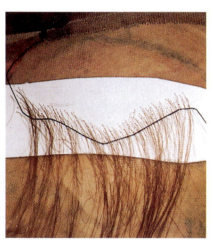

Knotting (continued)

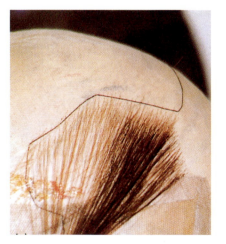

The front edge hairline completed and ready for filling in with main hair

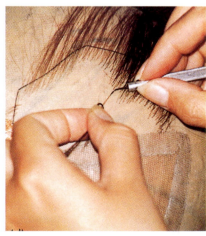

The completed front edge being checked for softness of hairline before continuing with knotting

Other postiche work

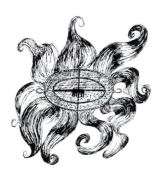

A chignon: view from underneath to show the foundation with loops and a comb to attach the piece to the head

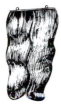

A marteau with hoops

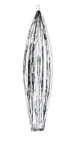

A switch

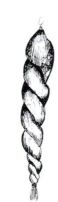

A coiled switch

A pincurl

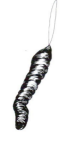

A ringlet

Extra pieces of postiche can be added to a wig, or to the natural hair when a wig is not required.

- **Bandeaux wigs** or **cape wiglets** Can be knotted or wefted postiche. This kind of hairpiece is used in turning a short hairstyle into a long one. It is held in position by a band, leaving the real front hair showing. It can be any length at the back.

- **Chignons** Knotted or wefted postiche, worn between the crown and the neck. They are good for adding fullness, height and shape.

- **Double-loop clusters** Wefted postiche made by winding and sewing onto a cord and finished with loops at each end. They are attached to the head with sewn-on combs and used to provide a cluster of curls.

- **Fringes** or **frontal pieces** Wefted or knotted postiche, used on the front of the head.

- **Hidden comb** A bunch of curls attached to a hidden comb. The technique is also known as *top knots*. These may be knotted pieces, but are usually wefted. The weft is made on two silks and a wire which, when folded and sewn, forms a very pliable foundation piece.

- **Marteaux** Pieces of weft folded together. They are attached to the hair by means of combs or sewn loops. They are useful for adding a wave, when required.

- **Pincurls** Small pieces of weft, sewn into various curl shapes. They are useful in adding to the hairstyle when dressed.

- **Ringlets** Larger curls, also used for dressing into a finished style.

- **Semi-transformations** Smaller pieces, also used to add length to the existing hair.

- **Swathes** Made from two marteaux, sewn end to end. They are used for encircling the head.

- **Switches** Lengths of weft wound spirally around tailcord. They can be coiled, plaited and twisted and used in a variety of ways.

- **Torsades** Coiled pieces of postiche. They look attractive when added to the hair.

- **Toupees** Knotted hairpieces, made to cover bald areas of the head. They are used extensively in TV and film on male actors and chosen to match the natural hair.

- **Transformations** Hairpieces, either wefted or knotted, worn to add length or bulk to the existing hair. They are often used on men for period work.

- **Wigs** The largest postiche items, covering the entire head of hair.

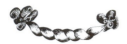

A torsade with curled ends

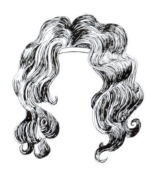

A bandeau wig

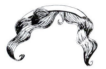

A frontal piece attached to a headband

Weft work

Weft work is the weaving of hair in the manufacture of postiche. The hair is interwoven onto silks, cotton thread or wire; interweaving at the root ends forms lengths of weft. The weft is folded, spirally wound, or sewn onto a *mount* or base. Wigs made in this way are known as *weft wigs* and many other pieces of postiche use woven or weft work.

Weft wigs and pieces are less expensive than hand-knotted pieces, although the quality of the finish is not suitable for TV and film. Weft work is useful for adding to natural hair to provide extra bulk and length in period hair work.

Activity – Visiting a wig company

Each wig company has a staff who specialise in the various aspects of wigmaking and wig dressing. Make-up artists spend much time there, attending fittings and chatting to other make-up artists and actors they know.

It is a good idea as a student make-up artist to visit a wig company. Here you can gain an insight into the making of postiche work from start to finish.

Wigs and hairdressing in the studio

Equipment

- Brushes
- Combs
- Heated rollers
- Tongs
- A hairdryer
- A malleable wig block
- A chin block (540 mm or 560 mm)
- A bench clamp or stand
- Galloon
- T-pins
- Long pins
- 'Short white' pins (small)
- Sectioning clips, pins and grips
- Acetone (be careful: this can be 'rough' on the lace)
- Cleaning solvent
- Surgical spirit (good for removing spirit gum)
- An artist's stipple brush or toothbrush

- An old sable make-up brush (for applying spirit gum and for applying surgical spirit to the lace to loosen it from the skin when removing wigs or facial hair)
- Spirit gum
- A damp cloth or powder puff
- A piece of silk or a piece of chamois leather
- An assortment of hairnets and stocking tops
- Crepe hair
- Heated tongs and a heater
- Moustache tongs (small)
- Hairspray
- Plastic spray

Cutting and styling the postiche

When the wig or other hairpiece has been made, it is pinned onto a malleable wig block and the hair is cut and styled in the required shape. The type of setting will depend on the period or fashion. This will have been discussed during the fittings and the wig dresser should have sketches, photographs and notes supplied by the make-up artist or hairdresser.

Postiche work is usually wet-set on rollers and placed in a special oven to dry slowly for several hours, often overnight. It is then brushed out and dressed in the desired style. For wig styles that are flat, such as the finger waving which was in fashion in the 1930s, the wig is set with the fingers and placed in the oven to dry in the same way.

Protecting the postiche

When the postiche arrives from the wig company it will already have been dressed and be ready to put on the artiste's head. It will come packed in tissue paper in a large wig box. On the lid will be the date of delivery, the name of the artiste, the name of the make-up artist and the name of the production company which has bought or hired the postiche.

Maintaining a wig

At the end of the first day's shoot, after it has been removed, the wig will need re-dressing and the hair lace will need cleaning. Once the lace has been cleaned, the wig should be placed on a wig block to keep its shape. Thus, the make-up artist or hairdresser must clean the wig when it gets dirty. She must then attach it to a block and restyle it, either returning it to the way it was or dressing it into a different style, according to the production requirements. Maintenance can therefore be divided into three areas: *cleaning*, *blocking* and *dressing*. Wigs can be *built up*, using added hairpieces.

Cleaning postiche

Whether the postiche is made from human or **synthetic hair**, it must be cleaned regularly and carefully. How often will depend on how long the wig or piece has been worn. If the wig is being used every day for weeks at a time, it is generally necessary to clean it at the end of each week.

Cleaning must be carried out with great care, so as not to damage the foundation and loosen the knotted hair or weft. Real-hair postiche should be cleaned in a recommended hair-cleaning solvent. Never use sharp combs, which can damage the foundation. Never use shampoo and water, as these cause tangling and loosening of the hair knots.

Cleaning real-hair postiche

Equipment and materials

- hair-cleaning solvent
- large bowl (porcelain, glass or metal – not plastic)
- wig block

1 Make sure the room is well ventilated – open a window, as the fumes from hair-cleaning solvents are as obnoxious as those from house paint.

2 Pour the hair-cleaning solvent into a large porcelain, glass or metal bowl. *Do not use a plastic bowl*: the chemicals in the cleaning solvent will melt the plastic.

3 Place the postiche in the cleaner until the base and hair are immersed. Leave for several minutes.

4 Move the wig or hairpiece around the bowl; then lift it up, allowing the liquid to drain back into the bowl.

5 When the liquid has finished draining off, shake the piece gently and hang it somewhere until the cleaning liquid has evaporated. If the weather permits, hang it outside in the open air.

6 When dry, place the postiche on the block, ready for setting, blow-drying, tonging or applying heated rollers.

Cleaning synthetic hair postiche

Shampoo can be used on synthetic hairpieces, as can *fabric conditioners* (such as Comfort).

Equipment and materials

- shampoo
- conditioner
- bowl
- towel
- wig block (covered with plastic)
- rollers, if required
- hairnet

1 Add shampoo to a bowl of lukewarm water. Make sure that the water is not too hot: extreme heat can damage the pre-formed curl in the hair.

2 Move the hairpiece gently in the water.

3 Rinse it in cold water.

4 Rub a conditioner, such as a fabric conditioner, into the hairpiece.

5 Hold the piece to let the water drain off into the bowl, then pat it with a towel and place it on a malleable wig block covered with plastic (to protect the block).

6 Set the hair with rollers or allow it to dry naturally, as required. The block, with a hairnet placed over it, can be placed in a warm airing cupboard or under a hooded hair dryer.

7 Most modern fibres can be set and blow-dried, or styled using hot tongs and heated rollers, but care should be taken: some artificial hair will be damaged by too much heat.

Equipment and materials

- small bowl (glass or enamel)
- towel, tissue or paper towel
- brush (toothbrush, sable make-up brush, or stipple brush)

Cleaning the hair lace on a lace-fronted, real-hair wig

At the end of the day, when the wig has been removed, the hair lace will need cleaning as it will have spirit gum and make-up on it. Surgical spirit is good for removing the spirit gum, as are **acetone** or methylated spirits. A toothbrush, sable make-up brush or stipple brush may be used to apply the spirit; the brush chosen must have hairs that are stiff enough to do the job properly.

1 Pour the spirit into a small glass or enamel bowl.
2 Place the hair lace of the wig onto a clean towel, soft tissue or paper towel.
3 Dip the brush into the spirit and tap it gently onto the wig lace, forcing the dried up spirit gum and make-up to go *through* the lace and onto the material below. Use a gentle but firm tapping motion. Be careful not to be too harsh, or the delicate lace will tear.
4 When the lace is clean, place the wig on the block, ready for blocking and setting.

Equipment and materials

- malleable block and stand
- blocking pins
- galloons
- 'short white' pins

Blocking the wig

1 Set up the malleable block and **wig stand** and carefully centre the wig in position on the block.
2 Make sure that the hairline at the front is in position. Check that the hairline in front of the ears is the same length on each side of the wig.
3 Use large blocking pins – **t-pins** – to secure the wig at the earpieces and at the corners of the nape area at the back of the wig.
4 Cover the lace front with galloon to reinforce the hair and protect the lace from being torn. Use small pins known as 'short whites', which minimise stress on the lace. Place the pins in a triangular pattern along the tape. Run the tape around the front hairline from ear to ear. Do not place any tension on the lace itself, only on the tape. Fold the tape to suit the shape of the hairline.
5 If the wig still feels loose, add long pins at the back of the wig until it feels secure on the block.

The wig is now ready for dressing.

Blocking a hair-laced wig

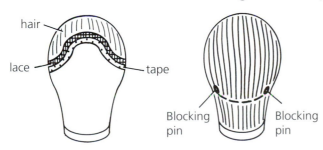

Put wig on from front to back: make sure that it is central

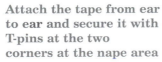

Attach the tape from ear to ear and secure it with T-pins at the two corners at the nape area

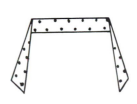

Tape down the lace, securing the tape with small pins in this pattern

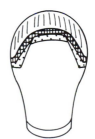

The wig is blocked and ready to be dressed

Dressing postiche

Equipment

When dressing postiche you will need the following equipment:

- Hairdryers – hand and hood types
- Tongs
- Crimpers
- Flat irons
- Heated rollers
- Setting rollers
- Various hairnets
- Clips, of various sizes
- Pins, of various sizes
- Grips, in various colours (matt if possible)
- Hairbands
- Haircombs
- Scissors
- Combs, including tail, setting, clubbing, and other types
- Brushes, including bristle, vent, half-round, round and other types
- Gels
- Mousses
- Sprays
- Water spray
- Toupee tape
- Spirit gum

Wig blocked and set in finger waves and pin curls

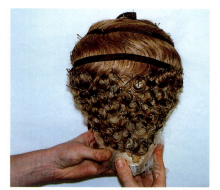

Back view

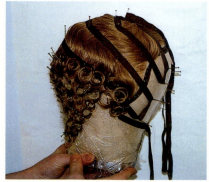

Side view

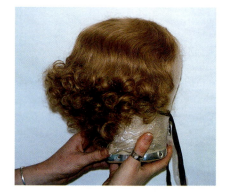

Dressed pit

Equipment and materials

- malleable block
- comb
- wig tape
- tail comb
- pins (large)
- hairnet

Finger waves

Finger waves were extremely fashionable in the 1930s. The technique of finger waving consists in moulding the wet hair into S-shaped movements using the fingers and a comb. Finger waving a wig is carried out as follows:

1 Block up the wig and spray down the hair. Be careful not to get the lace or the malleable block too wet.

2 Keeping with the root direction of the hair, make the first 'wave' of the hair by combing the hair from the roots.

3 Pinch the 'crest' of the wave between two fingers and comb the rest of the hair in the opposite direction.

4 Move your fingers down to pinch the next 'crest', then comb the rest of the hair, again in the opposite direction. Try to keep the waves an even width. Use your fingers as a guide – two fingers are about 30 mm.

5 Work in circles around the parting, taking the waves around the head until you reach the occipital bone. At this point continue with reverse pincurls, barrel curls, or pincurls set into the centre.

6 Secure the finger waves by applying wig tape across the 'dip'of the wave. Use a little tension and insert pins along the tape.

7 Place the block in a warm place to dry thoroughly.

It will help if you remember the following points:

- The hair should be combed thoroughly to rid it of any tangles.
- Use warm water to wet the hair and comb it on the slant backwards.
- Keep the hair wet (but not dripping) during the waving.
- Take care with the parting: it must be perfectly straight. Pin a tape along the parting to keep it neat, but do not place pins through the parting.
- For short hair, make shallow rather than deep waves.
- For a soft and natural look it is best to avoid deep waves, as these can look too hard.
- Short hair at the front of the wig can be curled separately.
- This gives a soft effect to the waves around the face and forehead.

Complete the dressing out as follows:

1 After removing the block from the oven or warm place, allow it to cool for a few minutes.

2 Using a tailcomb, lift up a thin layer of the hair along the parting. Backcomb the hair strongly near the roots, gradually lessening the backcombing as you work towards the points.

3 Continue making divisions and backcombing until the entire wig has been worked on.

4 Comb softly over the top to smooth the hair down and push or press the waves into position. Try not to comb out too much of the backcombing.

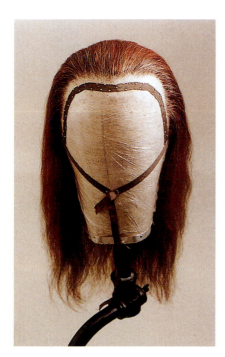

A wig blocked and ready for setting

Tip

In an emergency a wig can be dressed and waved very quickly using methylated spirits or cologne in place of water. This saves on the drying time, but it is just a standby method.

Equipment and materials

- clamps
- section clips (long)
- hairclips (small)
- hair dryer
- comb
- setting lotion, gel, mousse or emulsion (if required)

Equipment and materials

- heated rollers
- false hair (if required)
- brush and comb
- hairgrips
- hairpins
- tailcomb
- gel
- eyelash glue

5   Use one or two large pins to hold the waves down at the edges.

6   Leave the hair at the parting raised: hair on the head does not naturally grow flat from the parting.

7   Adjust the final shape, place a hairnet over the wig and return the wig to the oven or warm place for about 30 minutes.

8   Do not comb out the wig afterwards: this would remove the backcombing and leave the wig looking too flat. The top layer of hair only can be combed smooth.

Finger waving *natural hair* is a somewhat different process:

1   Make the finger waves as before, but secure them with clamps or long sectioning clips. Form any pincurls using small hairclips.

2   Place a net over the set and seat the artiste under a hooded hair dryer.

3   Do not backcomb during the final dressing out, as you would with a wig. Natural hair can be combed and pushed into position very easily, especially if the hair is finger waved with setting lotion, gel, mousse or emulsion whilst still wet.

Beehives and bouffants

Beehives and bouffants were fashionable in the 1960s. They can be created with or without false hairpieces, depending on the artiste's own hair. They can also be filled out with crepe hair.

1   First plan your beehive shape.

2   If you are using partings, set the hair in heated rollers.

3   Prepare any false hair if required.

4   Brush out the hair and backcomb it where you want the most height. Leave free any sections to be pulled over the bulk, kiss-curled or tonged. Keep most of the hair around the hairline smooth so that the final effect is sleek.

5   Make an anchor of grips down the centre of the back of the head. Smooth the hair from the right to the left.

6   Fold over the hair from the left and coil it round, securing it with hairpins. Keep the 'fold' very tight in the nape area. Add more pins as you work up the fold, securing the hair and covering the line of grips.

7   Coil round the backcombed hair on the crown to make the desired shape; fix this with pins.

8   Check the shape in the mirror and 'tease' it with a tailcomb to change the shape slightly if necessary.

9   Gel flat any pieces to be left out in the front.

10 Any small, wispy sections of hair can be pincurled and attached to the cheeks with eyelash glue. Tong any other pieces of hair that you want to leave loose.

For added height or a different shape, use crepe hair or a hairpiece. Wigs also can be set into beehives: a similar method is used on wigs to create an eighteenth-century look.

Building up a wig

Block your wig and begin to create a pre-planned shape. Then make a 'beehive', keeping it as flat as possible at the nape. To attach another hairpiece, make a pincurl base with hairgrips crossing over one another to form a cross. Attach the piece to the pincurl base, then work it in with the rest of the hair. Crepe hair also can be added – use it sparingly and secure it with hairpins. Extra pieces can be used for rolls, curls or tendrils.

Chicken wire can be used for a frame. Hair can be sewn into this with needle and thread, or attached with grips. Likewise, for extra bulk, crepe hair can be wrapped in netting before being secured to the wig. As much hair as you like can be added, but it must be secured well. Take care that the extra weight is not too uncomfortable for the artiste to wear. Refer to your design and don't attach more hair than is necessary.

Equipment and materials

- hairpiece
- hairpins

Hairpieces

Hairpieces add length and fullness. They may be attached as follows:

1   First assess the size and weight of the piece.
2   Make a pincurl base, either in the natural hair on the person's head or on the wig, as appropriate.
3   Attach the hairpiece to the pincurl base with hairpins. Hook a pin through the loop of the piece, pinching the pin together as you do this so that when you let it go it springs out and grips the surrounding hair.
4   Secure the hairpiece with more pins, making sure that they 'grip' into the pincurl base.

Equipment and materials

- parting piece
- toupee tape (if required)
- hairpins

Parting pieces

A parting piece is attached at the centre of the hair. Always look at the piece first, however, and place it on the head in different positions in order to find out where it looks best.

1   Make pincurls on the head with the natural hair to the side of the lace of the parting piece. If there is no hair, as on a balding man, toupee tape can be used.
2   Attach the piece with hairpins, weaving them in and blending them with the natural hair for a result that looks natural.

This method can be used for toupees and for any area of the head. The hair can be styled as required.

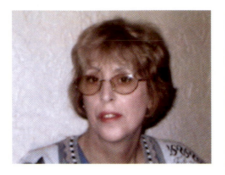

Marian Wilson

Case Profile
Marian Wilson, Wig maker

How long have you been working in the industry?
Thirty-five years.

How did you get into it?
From working in all departments in the theatre, I was drawn naturally to the wig department at the Royal Shakespeare Company. I was very lucky to be trained by them and have never looked back.

Who or what has been your most significant project?
After all these years that's very difficult to say. I like changing characters from young to old, such as Richard Dreyfuss in *Mr Holland's Opus*; *The Saint* where Val Kilmer played an old man; and fantasy films such as *Leprechauns*. Also recently I have worked on a 1950s and 1960s film, *Ali*.

What do you enjoy most about your work?
Not knowing what the next job will bring and not working just with hair but anything that will get the result you are looking for – from horsehair to wool.

And least?
Every job becomes repetitive at times. Looking at a design and thinking 'that would be fun' sometimes isn't when you have made 20 or more.

What advice would you give to people trying to get into this area of work now?
Learn your craft well. Never say you know it all. I'm still learning. And be willing to listen to others, especially artists, about how they see a character. They are the ones who are in the public eye, not you.

Attaching the wig

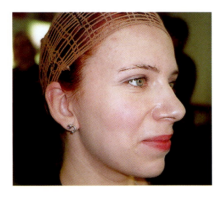

Preparing the head

Equipment and materials

- hairgrips
- stocking or hairnet
- hairpins
- gel or soap

Before attaching a lace-fronted wig to the head, carefully remove the tape and pins in order to detach the wig from the block.

Preparing the head

1 Use grips to pincurl the natural hair – two on the crown and one on either side of the head, forming anchors.
2 Wrap the remaining hair around the head.
3 Put stocking or hairnet on the head. Fix it with hairpins.
4 Gel or soap short hairs around the hairline.

If the wig has a parting, match the hair to it by parting it in the same way.

Attaching a wig to very short hair

When the artiste's hair is very short it is hard to make pincurls. Instead, therefore, use tiny rubber bands to secure the hair in very small tufts all over the head at the crown, nape and front hairline.

Tip

Take care that stray natural hairs do not prevent the wig lace from sitting flat to the head.

Attaching a wig to long hair

If the artiste has very long, thick hair, it is not possible to pincurl it flat. Instead, the hair should be wrapped around the head as flat as possible and covered with a hairnet or stocking top. Pins and grips can be used to secure it firmly.

Placing the wig

1 Hold the back of the wig with both hands and slide the wig front over the forehead.

2 Place one finger at the front of the lace to hold it in place, then pull down the back of the wig until it fits smartly on the head.

3 Holding the wig firmly on each side of the head (using the open palms of the hands), slide the wig front back until you reach the desired hairline.

4 Comb back any stray hairs, under the lace or away from the front of the wig.

Attach the lace to the head just in front of the natural hairline so that the hair growth does not appear to be too far down on the forehead.

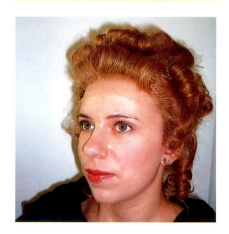

Placing the wig

Equipment and materials

● spirit gum adhesive
● damp cloth (muslin or milk)

Fixing the lace

1 Roll back the edge of the lace a little and apply spirit gum adhesive to the forehead in three spots.

2 With your fingertip, make the gum tacky.

3 Roll the lace back over the adhesive, pressing the edge onto the head with a damp cloth (muslin or silk).

Removing the wig

Equipment and materials

● surgical spirit
● small brush
● scissors
● mild mastix-removing liquid or cream
● pad of tissue, towel, or wad of cottonwool
● make-up cleansing milk or cream
● astringent or toner
● moisturiser

Always take great care when removing a wig or hairpiece with hair lace. You must not damage either the actor's skin or the lace itself.

Method: wigs with lace

1 Loosen the lace by applying a little surgical spirit on the brush to its edges.

2 Hold the tissue pad in the other hand, below the lace, so that any drops from the brush trickle onto the pad and not into the actor's eyes.

3 Continue gentle dabbing at the lace where it has been stuck down.

4 When the adhesive has softened, the lace may be lifted from the skin at the edges and rolled back to remove any remaining adhesive.

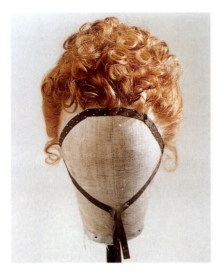

A dressed wig ready to be attached to the head

5 Remove the hairpins attaching the wig to the head.

6 Lift the wig off from behind, holding it carefully at the sides: pull it gently forward and off the head.

7 If it is a man's wig, detach the hairgrips from the anchor points on the crown and sides. If it is a woman's wig, remove the stocking or net and then remove the hairgrips on the head.

8 If the natural hair is so short that you used tiny rubber bands as anchor points, the simplest course is to cut them off carefully with scissors.

9 Remove any remaining spirit gum on the face using mild mastix remover.

10 Cleanse, tone and moisturise the skin to remove the make-up.

11 Brush through the hair to restore the artiste's normal hairstyle.

Method: wigs without lace

Remove these in the same way as wigs with lace (above), but without the surgical spirit and mastix remover.

Temporary colourings

Temporary colourings are often used in film and television to alter the colour of the natural hair or postiche. They can be used, for example, to disguise and cover white and grey hair and so make the person look younger, or to paint in white and silver hair and so make the person look older. They are also used to create exciting fashion effects.

Types of temporary colourings

There are many different types of temporary colourings. Here are the best known:

- **Coloured hair lacquers** These are sprayed onto the dried, dressed hair. They can be obtained from specialist theatrical make-up shops in a wide range of colours. They wash out easily.

- **Cosmetic hair-colouring liquids** These are available from theatrical make-up shops, packaged in bottles or wands (similar to mascara wands). The best way to use them from the bottle is to pour some into a dish and paint it onto the hair with a small make-up brush. The wand can be used directly onto the hair with its own applicator.

- **Gels and mousses** These are available in a limited range of colours and are easy to use straight onto the hair. They colour and condition the hair, and give extra 'hold'.

- **Hair colour crayons** These can be used directly on the dressed hair. They are useful for colouring in hair around the temples, or for filling in a bald patch on the head.

- **Hair colour creams** These are available from good specialist make-up shops. Packaged in small pots, they look like any other make-up creams. They are usually available in pink or light yellow and are painted onto individual hairs to neutralise dark hair before applying the chosen colour. They are generally used before putting ageing streaks of white, cream and silver at the front hairline. Without the cream neutralising colour, very dark hair always looks blue when streaked with cream, white or silver.

- **Hair colour setting lotions** These are applied to towel-dried hair and used to set the hair. They wash out easily.

- **Hair colour sprays** Available in liquid or powdered forms, these are also for use on the dried, dressed hair. They too wash out easily.

- **Hair gel glitter** This comes in a tube. It can be used on the hair or the skin. Colours are iridescent, giving strong effects under lights.

- **Hair glitter** This is available in loose form to sprinkle in the hair for a sparkling, glittering or twinkling effect. Though much of it is usually gold or silver, other colours are available. Glitter is tricky to control and goes everywhere, but it is good for adding glamorous effects to hair.

'Breaking down' effects

Very often a scene may require an actor to have his or her hair dirtied or made wet. The make-up must take account of the type of dirt – whether dusty or muddy, for instance – and the effect must look realistic.

Materials for dirtying the hair

- **Powders** Dark brown, grey or black powders are used for dry-looking dirt, such as coal dust.
- **Fuller's earth** is also useful for dirt.
- **Greasepaint** provides a greasy, matted effect.
- **Coloured hair-lacquer sprays** are useful for spraying on dark colours to 'break down' blonde hair.

Making the hair look wet

This is usually achieved using a *spray bottle* filled with water. The hair is sprayed before each 'take', and care must be taken to ensure that the continuity is maintained. Because sets and locations are so expensive, the order in which the production is filmed makes the most economical use of them. This seldom follows the order of the storyline. When filming rain scenes, therefore, it is always advisable to take a Polaroid photo of the actor's hair. The interior scene moments later, when the character comes in out of the rain, may actually be filmed several days later.

'**Breaking down**' effects add considerably to the realism of a scene. Co-operation is needed between the make-up and costume departments to achieve the degree of dirtiness required.

For casualty effects, 'blood' used on the hair should be of the washable kind: it will otherwise stain and be very difficult to wash out.

9

Facial hair

Introduction

Facial hair plays a significant part in changing men's appearances in productions for the theatre, television and films. It can assist in creating a character, and in portraying ageing. It is also important in period make-up work.

Postiche work for the face comprises *beards, moustaches, sideburns* and *eyebrows*. Beards, especially for opera singers, are sometimes made in three pieces, to ease the movement of the jaw. Exact measurements should be given whenever possible. A beard or moustache that does not fit properly can cause the actor great discomfort and can even hinder his speech and so spoil the performance.

Facial postiche cannot be hired, for reasons of hygiene and because it has only a short life. It needs to match or tone in with the colour of the wig or the actor's own hair. In the latter case, the postiche maker will need samples of the actor's hair, one from the top of the head and the other from the nape of the neck.

Facial hair is knotted onto lace – thicker for the theatre, very fine for film and TV work. As a make-up artist you will not generally be expected to make facial hairpieces, but you do need to understand the procedure in order to assess the quality of work when commissioning it from others. If as a student you want to learn the art of knotting, start with a moustache – don't tackle a full facial hairpiece at the first attempt.

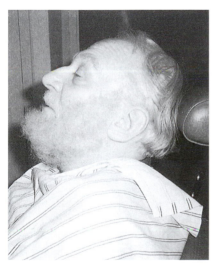

Facial hair: John Carter with his own moustache and an added full beard

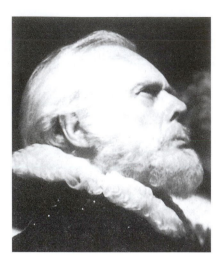

Marius Goring with his own hair
curled and added facial hair – a
moustache and a full beard

Historical background

Throughout history, facial hair has been very significant in men's appearances. The practices of trimming, shaving or partially shaving the face have often had an importance beyond vanity or mere habit. All over the world, shaving has at times taken on superstitious, religious or political significance.

Shaving has not always been voluntary. Occasionally, as in England at one time, shaving has been enforced by law. Likewise, when one area was invaded by people from another, the invaders would often impose their own practices.

Facial hairpieces

Making facial hairpieces

A moustache

Making a pattern

1   Place a piece of clingfilm on a flat surface. Cover it with adhesive tape to make it more solid. Cut out a V at the top, to allow a space for the nose.
2   Put this pattern on the person's face. With a make-up pencil, draw out the required shape.
3   Go over the pattern with more tape, to protect the pencil line. Use more tape to attach the pattern to the chin block.

Attaching the lace to the block

4   Place a piece of lace across the pattern and secure it around the edge of the shape using small pins.
5   Pin the lace as tautly as possible over the pattern. This makes it easier to apply pressure on the hair whilst knotting and thus to achieve tight knots. Stretch the lace evenly so as not to distort the direction of the line of holes.
6   The moustache pattern should be clearly visible through the lace. Make sure it is not off-centre on the block: the moustache pattern should be dead straight.
7   Place the block in the wooden box so that you can work on it comfortably.

Knotting the hair

Use a knotting holder and hook to knot the hair. Be careful with these hooks; as with fish hooks, it is easy to hook them back into your skin.

Equipment and materials

For making facial hair
- beard black
- knotting hook and needle
- hair lace
- small bowl of water (to dip the hair into)
- drawing mats (to hold loose hair)
- loose hair (yak)
- black pins
- cradle (a wooden box in which the block rests whilst you are working)
- tongs and tong heater (for dressing the hair)

For taking measurements
- tape measure
- clingfilm
- clear adhesive tape
- eyebrow pencil (brown or black)

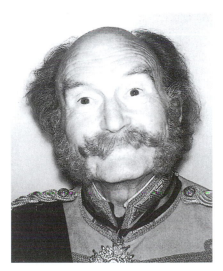

Maurice Denham with his own hair and added mutton chops and a moustache

8 Use yak hair for the moustache. Place the hair between two mats to keep neat. The mats have teeth on them: these should be turning towards you. Lay the hair over the teeth and push the mats together. As you pull the hair out, a bit at a time, the teeth will separate it.

9 Fold the hair in half and dip the doubled end in water. Continue to do this as you work.

10 Decide which way you want the hair to lie. If you want the hair to lie downwards, then knot upwards.

11 When you have completed the knotting of the moustache, trim the lace and hair to size and curl it with tongs into barrel curls.

12 Dress out the moustache to the finished style.

A beard

Measuring for a beard and taking a pattern for the beard follows the same procedure as for a moustache. When taking the pattern and applying the beard, the mouth should be open. Find someone whose chin you can practise on. For a production, of course, it would be the actor's. For TV and feature films the measurements and fitting must be exact.

Making a pattern

1 Put clingfilm across and under the mouth and up to the temples. Leave the nose uncovered, so that the artiste can breathe.

2 Cover it with adhesive tape, under the mouth.

3 Add tape underneath the chin.

4 Add tape from the sideburns to the jawline.

5 Add tape from the sideburns to the mouth.

6 Trim any excess clingfilm.

7 Use an eyeline pencil to draw the shape of the beard required. If possible, follow the pattern of the model's own beardline.

8 Cover the line with adhesive tape to protect it.

9 Place the pattern on the beard block.

10 If necessary, pad the block to the shape of the pattern.

11 To ensure a good fit, shape the lace for the beard into at least four pleats underneath the chin. 'Whip' or tack it into place with nylon thread or whipping nylon, using a hook.

Taking measurements

To make sure of the measurements, use a soft tape measure and send the details, as well as the pattern, to the postiche maker:

- the width of the sideburn (usually 25 mm)
- from the bottom of the mouth to the neck (usually 75 mm)
- from the sideburn to the point of the jaw (usually 75 mm)
- from the centre of the chin to the point of jaw (usually 100 mm)

A beard for an opera singer must be made longer than usual to compensate for the wide mouth movement during singing.

Making a moustache

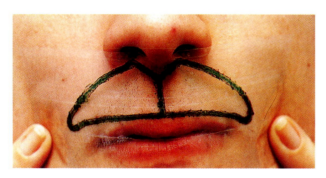

The moustache pattern is traced from the model's face using a soft eyebrow pencil and clingfilm reinforced with clear adhesive tape

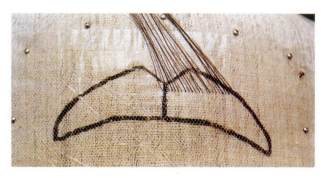

The resulting pattern is taped to a malleable block and a piece of lace is pinned tautly over the pattern, with the lines of holes running horizontally. One line of knotting has been completed on the first side. The hair is knotted in an upward direction and combed back down when completed

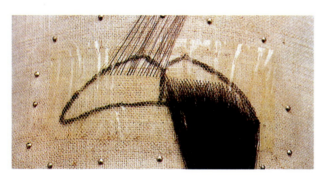

Most of the first side is now complete. One row of the opposite side has been knotted, showing that the hair is knotted in a different direction

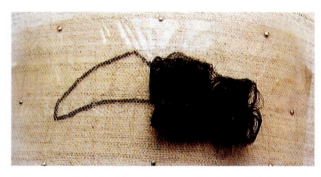

One completed side of a moustache, which has been curled into barrel curls using the small hot curling tongs

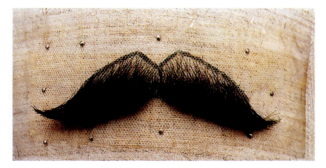

The finished dressing: both sides have been curled and the hair has been combed through, trimmed to the desired length and shaped into place with the tongs. A light coating of plastic spray will help to keep the dressing in place

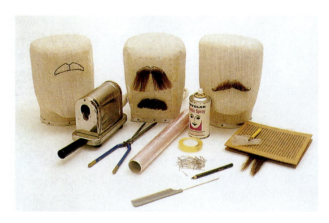

Facial hair equipment

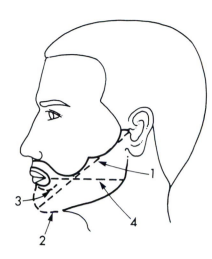

Measuring a beard: the dotted lines represent the measurements taken; the numbers show the sequence

---

Equipment and materials

- spirit gum remover or surgical spirit
- acetone
- tissues
- beard block
- pins

Equipment and materials

- spirit gum
- powder puff or cloth (damp)
- comb

Applying and removing facial hairpieces

Applying a moustache

1 Make sure that the skin is clean and free of grease. If you are unsure, use an astringent.
2 Using a brush, apply spirit gum to the skin.
3 Tap the spirit gum with your finger until it is tacky.
4 Place the moustache in position.
5 Use a damp powder puff or cloth to press the moustache down firmly. When the spirit gum is dry, comb the moustache into shape.

Removing the moustache

1 Use mild spirit gum (mastix) remover or surgical spirit. Dip a clean brush into the remover and stipple the edge of the lace to loosen it.
2 Slowly work around the edge until the moustache can be gently eased off.
3 Use remover to clean the rest of the spirit gum from the face.
4 Clean the moustache with acetone.
5 If ageing whitener has been used, soak the hair in surgical spirit for a minute and tissue dry it.
6 Pin the moustache to a beard block and re-dress it.

Applying a beard

1 Position the beard on the actor's face before applying spirit gum.
2 Apply spirit gum thinly to the skin on the chin area; tap the gum with your fingertip until it is tacky.
3 Adjust the position of the beard for the actor's comfort before pressing it down firmly with a damp cloth or powder puff.
4 If a full beard, turn back the beard at the sides of the face and apply spirit gum to the skin in the usual way.
5 When securing the beard in front of the ears, lift up the actor's own hair and stick the lace underneath.
6 Comb down the actor's own hair to hide the 'join'. If the colour is different, use a toning colour to blend the beard into the hair or wig.

Applying sideburns

Use the same method as you would when applying a beard – that is, sticking the lace under a small section of hair. On long productions and for big close-ups, it is best to cut or shave a small section of the actor's own hair after first lifting a section which can be allowed to blend over the adhered lace. There should be no visible gap between the sideburns or beard and the natural hair.

Equipment and materials

- beard block
- small moustache tongs (no. 1 irons)
- electric tong heater
- tissues
- pins
- lacquer (if required)
- plastic spray
- moustache wax (if required)

Equipment and materials

- lintless towel or muslin pad
- wig-cleaning brush or toothbrush
- surgical spirit

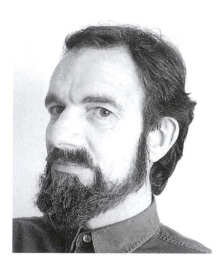

A beard and moustache

Tonging and dressing facial hairpieces

1 Pin the facial hairpiece on the beard block.
2 Heat a tong (small size). Test it on tissue to check that it is at the correct temperature.
3 Start at the top of the hairpiece, taking a section at a time, and tong the hair. Make sure that the hair is lifted at the roots.
4 Pin the dressed section out of the way.
5 When all the hair has been tonged, comb it into place. If necessary, spray it with hair lacquer.
6 Plastic spray, used sparingly, is useful in keeping an elaborately shaped moustache in place. **Moustache wax** can be used to pinch the ends of a moustache into a fine point.

Cleaning facial hairpieces

Facial hairpieces must have all the spirit gum removed from the lace before they can be dressed ready for using again. Acetone is the best solvent for cleaning hair lace.

1 Place the piece, lace down, on a lintless towel or muslin pad.
2 Use a wig-cleaning brush soaked in acetone to press the adhesive out of the lace and onto the towel. Use brush cleaner to remove any make-up, or stroke the lace gently with a muslin pad soaked in acetone. Do not brush the lace hard or you will tear it.
3 Using the stiff bristles of the brush, stipple onto the lace to force the surgical spirit through the holes of the net.
4 Move the piece to a clean area on the towel and repeat the process until the lace looks clean.
5 Allow the hairpiece to dry out thoroughly before re-dressing it.

A toothbrush can be used to clean the lace. Another way of cleaning lace, which is quicker and used in theatres, is to make a pad from cheap muslin folded around a flat wad of cottonwool which has been soaked in acetone. A similar pad, soaked in mild spirit gum remover, is used for cleaning the spirit gum from the actor's face.

There are also special creams for removing adhesives from the face. These are used by some make-up artists.

Applying facial hair directly to the skin

Instead of using hair knotted onto lace, another way of adding facial hair is to apply it directly to the face. An art in itself, this process has two great advantages. When facial hair is laid directly onto the actor's face it is impossible to tell that it is false, as there is no lace edge to conceal. Also, with the right tools and sufficient expertise, a make-up artist can create any style at a moment's notice when there wouldn't be enough time to commission or make the piece. The addition of laid-on hair is a skill with other applications, including the overlaying of hair on the edges of hair laces to change the shape of a hairpiece or to soften a hard-looking line.

Preparing the hair

The hair as received from the supplier is straight. In this condition it is very difficult to spread evenly, so to be able to spread and control it it is necessary to treat the hair first.

1   Crimp the hair with the no. 1 tongs.

Hackling the hair

1   Draw the hair through the teeth of the hackle to separate the different lengths.
2   Place these in the teeth of the hackle in order of the colours, very much like paint on a palette.

Mixing the hair

To achieve a natural effect with facial hair you need to mix several colours together. A head of hair, even of black hair, is made up of hair of several colours. Never lay a one-tone beard or moustache as this would look phoney.

By mixing hair carefully you will be able to achieve any of the colours and tones that occur in natural facial hair. Take care not to overmix the hair, however, or you will make only a nondescript colour – in this respect the process is very much like overmixing paint.

Equipment and materials

- hackle
- scissors
- comb
- curling tongs (no. 1 moustache irons)
- spirit gum
- brush
- acetone
- Vaseline
- loose hair (yak – black, dark brown, blond, red, white)
- electric tong heater

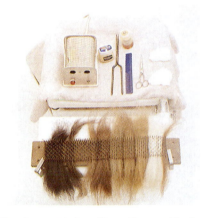

Equipment for directly applied facial hair

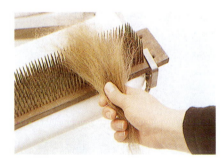

Hackling the hair

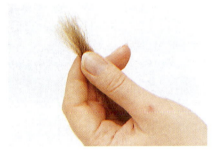

Hair held between the thumb and forefinger

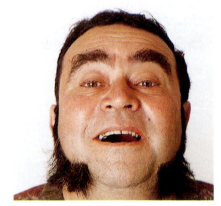

Side whiskers

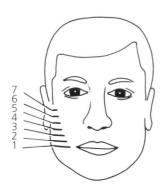

Laying hair for side whiskers

>
>
> **Tip**
>
> The correct way to hold the scissors is with the thumb and third finger. The bottom blade is held steady by the third finger; the upper blade, operated by the thumb, performs the cutting.

> **Tip**
>
> When laying hair for beards, start with mid-deep brown, then work through mid-brown to light brown, and use blond for the last few strands.

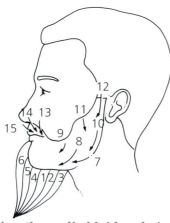

Directly applied laid-on hair: the arrows show the direction of growth; the numbers show the position and sequence of application

Laying the hair

A sidewhisker

Your equipment should be clean and laid out neatly.

1   First place a fine cutting comb under the man's own sideburns and lift them upwards to expose the skin underneath. Secure the comb in position by placing it over the top of the man's ear.

2   Using the brush, paint a thin layer of spirit gum onto the desired shape of the sidewhisker.

3   Wipe the scissors on the acetone pad, to remove any spirit gum, then wipe them on the Vaseline pad to coat the blades lightly. This helps to prevent the build-up of gum on the blades and should be repeated frequently during the process of the laying.

4   Now draw the hair from the hackle, holding it between the thumb and forefinger of the left hand if you are right-handed and the right hand if you are left-handed.

5   Taking the scissors in your other hand, spread the hair onto the gummed area by rolling the hair between the forefinger and thumb and lightly tap the ends of the hairs so that they adhere to the gum. Cut these hairs to the required length.

Note that you lay hair *starting from the bottom and working upwards*.

A beard and a moustache

For a beard the process is similar. Note that soft edges are produced by thinning out, and by using lighter coloured hair. Never make an actor look bland and dull by using one colour. With black beards, add a little white or red to give colour, interest and life to the character.

1   Apply spirit gum under the chin in the desired shape.

2   Draw the prepared hair from the hackle, applying it to the face as described above for sidewhiskers. Use the darkest colours underneath, fanning out the hair with the forefinger and thumb.

3   When it has adhered, cut the hair to the required length.

4   Mix in a lighter colour and keep applying a small section a time. Always mix some light hair into dark hair.

5   Work up towards the mouth, adding the lightest colours.

6   When a fairly large area has been covered, use a towel to press onto the hair firmly (for extra pressure, gently use your thumbs). This secures the hair and gets rid of the extra gum and the odd loose hairs.

7   Start to apply the moustache, section by section.

8   As you work up the side of the jaw, start thinning the top hairs out and use a lighter colour of hair.

9   When finished, use a large-toothed comb to comb gently through the beard and moustache.

10 Cut the hair into the shape required. Use eyebrow tweezers to remove unwanted hairs.

Equipment and materials

- heated tongs
- tissues
- comb
- scissors

Dressing out the beard and moustache

The laid-on beard and moustache need to be styled (dressed out):

1 Heat the **tongs**. Test the temperature on a tissue: if the tongs singe the tissue, wait until the correct temperature has been reached.

2 Use the hot tongs to dress the hair. Rest them on a comb held in the other hand, to avoid touching the face with the tongs. Start at the roots and, using the tongs, shape the beard.

3 Turn the underneath layers upwards.

4 Trim and style the beard to the shape you want. Bring hair down to cover any gaps.

Laying on a beard and moustache

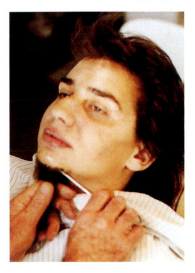

Applying loose hair under the chin

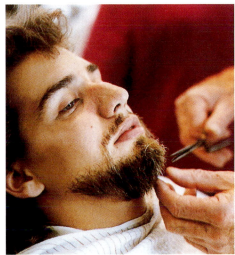

The hair has been applied and is trimmed into place, ready to be dressed with tongs

Hair stubble

Although it is possible for an actor to grow a short stubble by simply not shaving for a few days, it is often necessary to create one. Because filming is seldom in the same order as the storyline, continuity often demands that the actor be both clean shaven and unshaven in the same day's work. It might seem common sense to film his 'unshaven look' scenes first, but this is not always possible.

Although at a distance the look can be simulated with make-up, in tight close-up for feature films it is necessary actually to be able to see the hairs sticking out of the face.

Equipment and materials

- short cut-up real hair (3 mm long)
- piece of hair lace
- powder brush (soft)
- wax (**stubble paste**)

Applying the stubble

1 Spread wax thinly on the face, following the natural beardline.

2 Have some finely chopped hair (human hair is best) in a bowl. Place a small piece of hair lace (70–100 mm square) on the wax and press it on.

Applying beard stubble

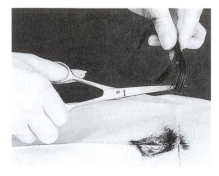

Cutting the hair finely, about 3 mm in length

3   Start at one side of the face, where the beardline begins, on a level with the ear. Dip the soft powder brush onto the prepared hair stubble so that it picks up the hair evenly on the tip of the brush. Stipple the brush onto the hair lace held against the skin. Use light movements to convey the hair through the lace, onto the wax below.

4   When you have finished, pull off the lace very carefully, leaving the hairs attached to the wax.

5   Move on to the next section, covering the entire beardline using the same method. The moustache and chin areas are the hardest to do.

6   If any small areas are missed, it may be necessary to apply more wax and go over these sections again. Tiny areas can be strengthened with dark greasepaint and a small pointed brush.

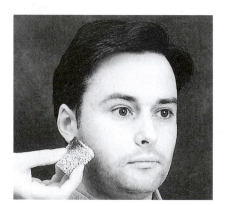

Darkening the natural beardline with greyish-blue greasepaint. The greasepaint is then powdered and a fine stipple wax is spread onto a small area of beardline

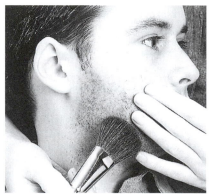

The hair lace is stretched across the skin and the loose hair stippled through the hair lace with a soft brush. The hair lace is then pulled away, leaving the hairs sticking out. This is repeated, a small section at a time, across the beardline

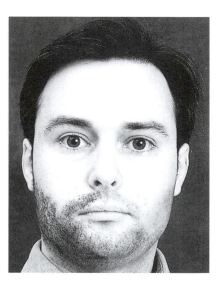

The final effect, showing the beardline completed on one side

Remember to take the growth down onto the neck under the chin, as far as the Adam's apple.

Another way of applying stubble is to darken the beardline with greyish-brown compressed powder. Then apply the wax on top and finish off by applying finely chopped wool crepe hair using a brush. This method is excellent for the stage and television, but in close-up shots for feature films it is ineffective. The hairs do not stick out from the face as they do when using hair lace.

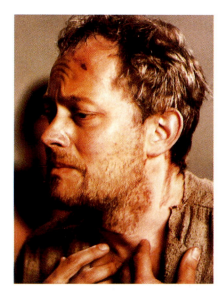

Facial hair, using six pieces, dirtied down: Michael Pennington in *Cymbeline*

Removing the stubble

1   To remove hair stubble, apply cleansing cream to the beardline and scrape off the hair and wax with a spatula or palette knife.

2   Finish off with normal cleansing, toning and moisturising, to restore the artist's face to normal.

10

Casualty effects

Introduction

By applying material directly to the skin and then shaping and colouring it, many special make-up effects can be achieved. The best known and perhaps the most impressive visually are *casualty injuries*. There are two stages:

1 Applying and building the material to create the effect.
2 Finishing the effect with colour and texture.

Planning the effect

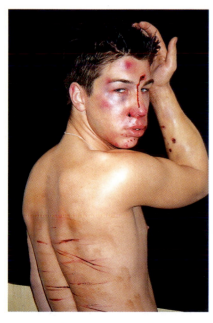

Victim of violent attack

Basic casualty effects are called for on many types of productions, ranging from medical documentaries, through drama, to horror videos. All of the materials used can be obtained from professional make-up suppliers, but many can be made by the make-up artist using kitchen ingredients. Thus, **latex**, **mortician's wax** and **plastic scar material** are specialist products used to build up three-dimensional effects on the skin, but most of the other materials can be found in food stores: **gelatine** powder, vegetable colourings, **glycerine**, petroleum jelly (from chemists), coffee granules, cereals, black treacle.

It is easy to get carried away when doing casualty make-up. Over-enthusiasm may result not only in 'over the top' effects but in effects that are difficult to reproduce. It is essential to be in control and to suit the effect to the production's needs. In a horror film it may be fine to go all the way, but restraint should be exercised in more realistic dramas. So before splashing on a lot of blood, remember that your design comes

Tip

Don't paint yourself into a corner. Stay in control. Always take notes.

first, and consult the director. However impressive or convincing the effect, the director won't thank you for creating a horrific slit throat for a prime time television series when children may be watching. These are the questions to ask before applying the make-up:

Wounds

1   How obtrusive is each wound to be?
2   What caused it?
3   How will it heal?
4   How can you repeat it?

Bullet wounds

1   What calibre was the gun?
2   From how close was the shot fired?
3   Is the casualty dead or alive?

Bruises

1   Where are the bruises to be positioned?
2   How old are they?
3   What caused them?

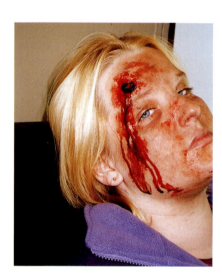

Facial wounds and blood

Equipment and materials

- Barrier cream
- 'Blood' – different brands and colours; running blood; congealed blood (black treacle or blue food colouring will help in darkening the blood)
- Spray containers
- Medicine bottle droppers
- Palette containing red, blue, yellow, green and black
- Greasepaints
- Scar plastic
- Latex
- Mortician's wax
- Sealer
- Spirit gum, spirit gum remover
- Vaseline, KY jelly, gelatine, glycerine
- Coffee granules
- Collodion
- Tear stick
- Black cotton
- Scissors

Water sprays

A *spray bottle* with a fine nozzle filled with water is useful for refreshing blood on wounds during fight scenes. It is also used on the hair to refresh hair gel and to reactivate it during the course of a day's shoot.

For heavy fight scenes the spray can be filled with half water and half glycerine to provide perspiration. If you put a fine layer of Vaseline on the actors' foreheads first, the mixed glycerine and water will adhere to the area and not dry too quickly.

Gelatine

Gelatine is very useful in casualty effects and can be applied directly to the skin. It can be coloured red to provide an excellent 'blood' which doesn't run. It is harmless to the skin and provides fast, effective results.

Basic recipe for direct application of gelatine

Equipment and materials

- gelatine powder
- glycerine
- water
- colouring (pancake scrapings, powder pigments, etc.)

1   Use equal amounts of gelatine powder and glycerine, plus water and colouring. Mix the gelatine and glycerine together and heat them gently in a saucepan on a stove, adding a small quantity of water at a time. (It is easier to add water gradually than to add gelatine.) Heat gently until the mixture has clarified.

2   When clear, add the colouring. Add a little more water until you are happy with the texture.

3   Test by putting some first onto a plate and then applying it to the back of your hand. *Be careful not to burn yourself.* The mixture should be warm enough to be liquid when it is applied, cool enough to be harmless to the skin and thick enough to set quickly.

Colouring effects

The gelatine can be coloured in advance, to give a flesh effect, for use as blood which stays in place or, using additional colour, as a burns effect. This can be achieved by adding food colouring – red, for a blood effect – into the gelatine mixture. It is also easy to colour the gelatine once it has been applied to the skin and become firm to the touch. Powdering and painting with watercolour paints on top produces a good effect. Other substances can be mixed in for added textural effects – dirt and gravel, even glass fragments, splinters, and so on. It will all wash off with soap and hot water.

Gelatine is easy to apply, using sponges, brushes or **modelling tools** to transfer the gelatine straight onto the skin. For a really firm hold you can use spirit gum on the skin before applying the gelatine on top. The beauty of using gelatine is that it is completely harmless to the skin and provides an excellent translucent look which is very effective.

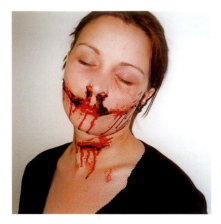

A gruesome knife wound known as 'The Chelsea Smile'

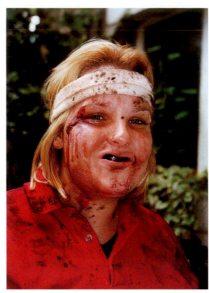

'Rugby player'

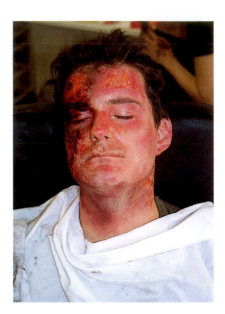

Third degree burns

Blood recipe
2 oz/62 g gelatine
2 fl oz/57 ml water
2 oz/62 g glycerine

Mix together in saucepan and gently heat until ingredients have dissolved. Add a few drops of red food colouring. To make darker add black food colouring. Brown could be added for a slightly different colour.

Keep in a flask for use later. A few seconds in the microwave will soften it up, if necessary. It can get very hot, so never put it directly onto someone else's skin.

Bread crumbs, rice crispies and cornflakes can be added to the blood to make good injuries.

Health and safety

Tip

The non-stain 'blood' available from specialist shops is excellent but expensive.

All the materials you use for special effects should be treated with respect. Some of the materials can be harsh and damaging to the skin. Always test them first on a less delicate area of the artiste's skin, such as the back of the hands. Before using spirit gum, latex or scar plastic on the face, apply a good barrier cream.

When removing the make-up, do so with care. Never rub and take plenty of time. Treat the other person's face as gently as you would your own.

An essential part of the learning process is that you should experience every make-up effect tried on yourself, as well as trying it on others. Only then will you realise what it feels like. Students should practise on one another before attempting make-up on a model or an actor.

Manufacturers' instructions for the use of their products must always be followed. The *COSHH 1988 regulations* (see page 5) provide requirements and guidance for the safe practice and storage of potentially dangerous substances.

Cuts and wounds with colouring

1 Apply congealed 'blood' with a modelling tool or dentist's scalpel. Shape the cut or wound.

2 Put *blushing gel* (or red gelatine) over the cut or wound to give more depth.

Raspberry jam and warmed red gelatine will produce a good effect. Face powder, talc or flour can be used as a thickening agent.

Grazed and dirty hands

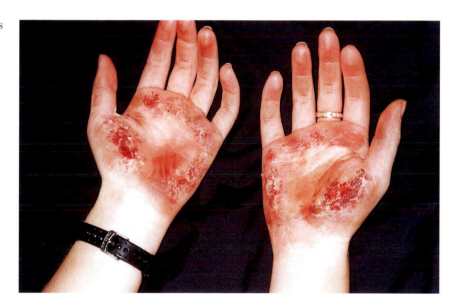

Deep wounds

Apart from changing the shape of the face, wax can be used for building up an area which can then be cut into for a deep cut or wound.

1 Spread the wax fairly thinly. Blend the edges as usual.

2 Cut into the wax with a palette knife or the end of a brush to make the required incision. Apply sealer.

3 When dry, colour the area to match the surrounding skin. Put red into the wound and finally a trickle of 'blood'.

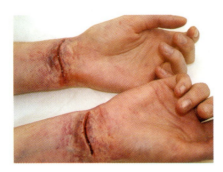

Slit wrists

Equipment and materials

- wax
- palette knife or brush
- sealer
- colouring
- 'blood'

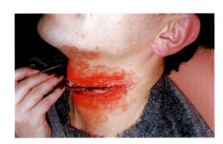

A slit throat

Equipment and materials

- greasepaint (red and brown)
- mortician's wax
- modelling tool
- sealer
- camouflage make-up (pink or red)
- powder puff
- cosmetic sponge
- palette knife
- scab material
- wound filler
- colouring
- coffee granules
- 'blood'

Slit wrists

1 Start with placing wax on the area that is to be slit.

2 Evenly distribute the wax so it blends with the skin.

3 Using flesh-toned greasepaints, paint the wax to create a more realistic look.

4 Place a slice in the wax using a plastic knife. Paint the wound area with bruise colours (blue, purple, red).

5 With a paintbrush, dab fake blood into the crease created by the slice.

The process takes around 30 minutes.

Slit throat

Before starting, think about what caused the wound: was it a serrated or smooth-edged knife? Think about the length, depth and shape of the cut.

1 Paint red and brown greasepaint onto the area of the wound.

2 Soften some mortician's wax in your hands and apply it to the wound area with a modelling tool. Keep to the natural shape of the neck and blend the edges well.

3 Build up the wax in the centre of the wound to the required depth.

4 When the shape is right, apply two coats of sealer, allowing the first coat to dry before painting on the second.

5 Paint pink or red camouflage make-up over the sealer to blend it with the surrounding natural skin tones. Powder.

6 Add more camouflage make-up, stippling on the colour with a cosmetic sponge and paying particular attention to camouflaging the edges of the wax. Bruising and redness can be added around the area at this point. Powder again.

7 Now, using a palette knife, slit through the wax with a smooth sweeping movement.

8 Very gently, pull back areas of the wax, according to the desired effect.

9 Fill the wound with fresh scab material, wound filler and raw-flesh colour.

10 Add some coffee granules.

11 Before the shoot, apply congealed and flowing 'blood'. Don't put on too much or the 'blood' will hide the wound make-up work you've done.

Case Profile
Christine Powers, Make-up and hair designer

How long have you been in the industry?

In excess of twenty years.

How did you get into it?

At 14 years old I wrote to the BBC to ask what I should do. Their advice was to go to the London College of Fashion and then make an application. At 19 I was accepted for training at the BBC.

What or who has been your most significant project?

A wonderful children's series called *Maid Marion and her Merry Men*. Written by and starring Tony Robinson, with every aspect of make-up, period, prosthetics and disguise. David Bell was the director, and it had a wonderful cast. It was the best organised and scheduled programme I have ever worked on.

What do you enjoy most about your work?

The amazing variety – no job is ever the same and you are always meeting new people.

And least?

It is a pain and pleasure industry. The hours can be very long. Broken engagements.

What advice would you give to people trying to get into this area of work now?

Determination and patience. Give any job a go, certainly at first. Have a life. I have had three sons and taken time out. You do not lose your way. There will always be work. With a life you cope better with your job and keep it in perspective.

Bruises and black eyes

A bruise can usually be created using paint only. The colours used are red, grey, purple, greenish-yellow and light cream or ivory and browns. The fresher the bruise, the redder it is; the older it is, the more yellow and brown it becomes. The stages of a bruise are as follows: red; reddish blue or dark purple; brown; paler brown; yellowish-green; yellow (in the last stages of healing). Colours can be dabbed on and then blended well or brushed and stippled. Make sure that the edges are soft and the colours blended away. Rub the colour in well.

For swellings, build up first with wax. Swellings look most convincing on bony areas such as the eyebrow bone.

Think about the rest of the face as well as the particular bruise. The victim might be bruised in other places and appear pale from shock. What is the situation? What caused the bruise?

Bruises should always look as though they have worked from the inside of the skin outwards; they must not look as if they were painted on. Think about the shape, the impact and the unaffected areas, as well as the 'age' of the bruise.

Never overdo the bruise (or any other casualty effect) for TV or film. If your critical eyes won't accept the effect as believable, the camera

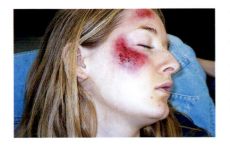

Bruising

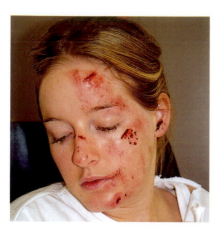

Scratches

Equipment and materials

- stipple sponge (coarse)
- grease (grey-brown)
- fine brush
- coffee granules
- 'blood'

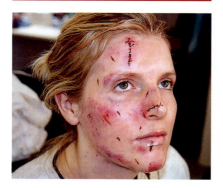

Stitched wounds

Equipment and materials

- black cotton
- scar plastic
- spirit gum
- colouring
- 'blood'
- scissors (sharp)
- Vaseline or oil

certainly won't either. You may have continuity to consider. If so, you must be able to match the bruise exactly the following day, or even weeks later. Before gleefully creating hideous scars and burns, think carefully. Remember: more is less. In some circumstances you will need to apply dirt and scratches around the bruise or scar.

One way to build up a bruise is to work in the main colours and then smear a thin coat of wax over the top. Although bruise palettes are good, it is better to learn to mix your own colours from a normal basic colour palette.

1   Create the darkest part of the bruise first. Blend the edges. Don't make the bruise look too neat or too like eye shadows.

2   The bruise should look shiny, so add some Vaseline at the last moment.

Scratches

1   Use a coarse stipple sponge with a little grey-brown grease. Draw it quickly across the face. The sponge will leave small lines which will act as realistic guidelines for your scratches.

2   With a fine brush, paint some 'blood' on different parts of the scratch marks. Add tiny dots of congealed 'blood', unevenly. (If the scratches look even they will not be convincing.)

3   Dot coffee granules here and there. Be subtle, or the 'scratches' will develop into severe cuts.

Stitched wounds

Although colourless adhesive strips are often used in casualty departments to bind wounds together, the old-fashioned stitches are still used in some circumstances. If a wound is irregular, the expertise of the stitching is of vital importance in helping the skin to knit together neatly.

1   Use black cotton (double thread). Calculate how many stitches you need. Tie double knots at about 25 mm intervals along the thread.

2   Cut between the knots, in the middle. Bend in the thread, halfway from the knot.

3   Use scar plastic in a very fine line to create a gather of skin. Quickly press the stitches into the plastic, before it dries. (If necessary, you can use spirit gum to stick them.) The knots should be stuck down at 12 mm intervals along the 'wound'.

4   Redden the area around the stitch line variably to look sore. With a fine black eyebrow pencil, draw in lines on either side of the cotton knots.

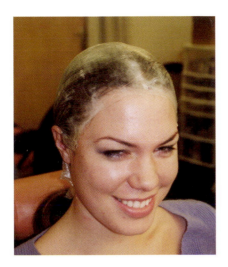

Burns
Before make-up

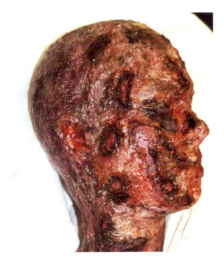

Burned to death
Make-up artist Shauna O'Toole.
Model Camilla Tew

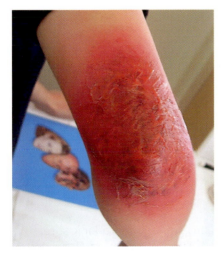

A second-degree burn

Put a small drop of congealed 'blood' at the base of several of the 'stitches'. With sharp scissors (do not use hairdressing scissors or they will be blunted), cut the long ends of the cotton neatly all the way along. Finally, add a little Vaseline or oil to give a shiny, stretched look to the area. (Sealer can be used instead.)

 Activity – Burn project

1 Make bald cap with cap plastic.
2 Melt gelatine.
3 Paint one layer of gelatine on the skin and place torn-up tissue directly on top. Follow by painting one more layer of gelatine on top of the tissue.
4 Using skin-coloured greasepaints, (peach, blues, and rose tones), paint the dried top layer of gelatine.
5 Rip random holes in the gelatine creating the raw skin look.
6 Around the rims of the holes use black greasepaint and deep red tones to scarcely colour the additional areas creating a burned, fleshy look.
7 Top the torn areas with a fake blood to create a fresh look.
The process takes around 1.5 to 2 hours.

Burns

As always, plan the effect. How was the burn caused? How old should it be?

- A *first-degree burn* is slight, usually causing redness and sometimes a small blister.
- A *second-degree burn* causes severe blisters. Remember when creating a second-degree burn to surround it with a first-degree burn.
- A *third-degree burn* will cause much more severe lacerations: the flesh may even be charred and black. Around this you should place second-degree burns and, towards the edge, first-degree burns.

Alternative techniques for a third-degree burn

1 Place a single layer of cleaning tissue – tear the shape, do not cut it with scissors – across the latex while it is still wet. Cover the tissue with another layer of latex.
2 For a charred flesh effect, add a small amount of cottonwool. Apply another layer of latex. When the latex is dry, spray the area with black hair colouring. When dry you can peel this back to the skin in bits: this will resemble charred skin.

3   Put some gelatine in a bowl or plastic bag and place it in a container filled with hot water. When the gelatine has melted – but make sure it isn't too hot – apply it to the burn to give a shiny, blistered effect. Let the gelatine form small droplets around the burn, like blisters. Alternatively, push Vaseline underneath areas of the latex.

You can apply make-up over all these products, but usually this is unnecessary. Vaseline, KY jelly or glycerine can also be used to give the shiny effect of blistered skin. Burn effects can make use of scar material, latex built up in layers, or gelatine. Scar material can be spread roughly and punctured when dry, with blood being pushed into the 'blisters'. Latex gives a shrivelled effect. Clear gelatine on top gives a watery, blistered look. The most severe part of the burn should have the greatest depth. Around this the effect should fade away, with blisters and redness.

Creating a burn with latex, tissue, gelatine and colouring

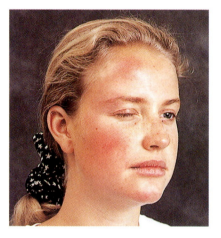

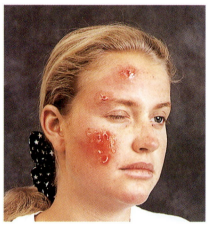

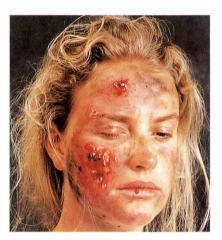

First-degree burn: red greasepaint was applied to the face

Second-degree burn: latex and tissue were applied to prominent areas with a modelling tool. For speed, the latex was dried with a hairdryer. When dry the latex was pulled to give a 'torn skin' effect. More redness was painted on and gelatine added for the blistering effect

Third-degree burn: black colouring, another layer of gelatine and black smudges (using black powder) have been added

Acne

Using a hairpin, place plastic scar material in tiny spots on the face to give the appearance of acne. Don't make the spots all the same size. Place them in clusters, particularly around the mouth and chin. You can add redness, or Vaseline on each one to make them look 'weepy'. Make the surrounding skin area look red and irritated.

Dirtying down

Dirtying down can be achieved using black and brown grease. The colour will be determined by the type of dirt needed, which in turn depends on the location – desert, swamp, forest, street, mine, and so on. Apply the grease using a natural sponge with holes it it.

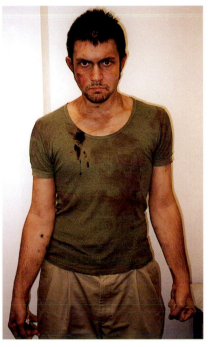

Dirtied down look

Head and face

1   Ask the artiste to frown and pull in the eyebrows. Apply brown grease over the wrinkles caused by frowning.
2   Put some grease around the nose and on the tip. Use a minimal amount and build it up.
3   Apply grease behind the ears, to the back of the neck, and under the chin; work into the neck creases and the ears.
4   If a darker effect is required, repeat lightly with black grease.

Hands

1   With a thin brush, put dark brown or black into the cuticles and rub around and under the nails.
2   Rub between the fingers and on the knuckles – in real life the creases always get dirty.

Dirtying down and blood

1   Dark brown grease or pancake applied using a damp natural sponge (bath size) is excellent for achieving a fast natural look for dirt.
2   The large holes in the natural sponge prevent the make-up from going on too evenly. Repeat with black pancake, stippled all over and rubbed in well to add emphasis.
3   Pay attention to the neck area.
4   Remember to discolour and put brown or black under the fingernails and around the cuticles.
5   Fill two spray bottles, one with 'blood', the other with water. When the action is to be filmed, first spray on 'blood', then water, at the last minute.

Tooth blacking and dirtying

Teeth can be blacked out with **tooth enamel** to give the appearance, from a distance, that they are missing. Though this works well on stage, the blacking out is obvious in film or television close-up. Enamel can also be used to 'break down' the teeth, making them appear dirty and irregular.

As with all make-up, use enamel sparingly. Often it is sufficient to paint small patches onto the teeth, close to the gums. The best approach is to paint the teeth first with a yellow nicotine colour, then to dot black on once the yellow has dried.

Equipment and materials

- grease (brown)
- pancake (black)
- natural sponge
- spray bottles (with 'blood' and with water)

Equipment and materials

- tissue
- small brush
- tooth enamel (nicotine yellow and black)

Anything placed in the mouth is unpleasant for the actor and such techniques should be used only with great caution. Few actors are comfortable about using tooth enamel, especially if they have expensively capped teeth. In any case, the added enamel quickly wears off with eating and drinking, so it is tricky to maintain during filming.

1 Dry the tooth with a tissue.
2 Using a small brush, paint nicotine-coloured tooth enamel onto an area of the tooth close to the gums.
3 Rub this gently with your fingertip so that it looks worn in. Leave it to dry.
4 To emphasise the dirtiness, add a tiny dot of black enamel.

Removing the enamel

Put a small amount of surgical spirit on a cotton bud. Rub this over the tooth to remove the added enamel.

Scars

Scars may be new or old, inverted or protruding. As ever, you need to plan the effect according to the needs of the production.

Scars may be made using special plastic, available in several brands and packaged in tubes which make it easy to apply. The work is quick and the results realistic. Alternatively, latex can be used – any type will do.

You can even use the adhesive made for false eyelashes, as this too is made of latex. Although it is desirable to have planned thoroughly and to be well organised, every professional make-up artist has had experiences of improvising effects at the last minute. The unexpected is part of the fun of the business, and some directors are a continual challenge to one's ingenuity.

An old scar: Nastassja Kinski in the film *Revolution*

1 Apply barrier cream and rub it in well.
2 Draw a line where the scar is going to be, using scarlet or crimson lake greasepaint or pencil.
3 Apply scar plastic or latex along the line, directly from the tube or with a modelling tool.
4 Before the material dries, shape it quickly using the tool.
5 For a *new scar*, paint crimson lake around the edges in an uneven way. Blend a little scarlet red as well, to look sore. Leave it shiny. For an *old scar*, paint brown around the edges and powder all over to give a faded effect.

Equipment and materials

- barrier cream
- modelling tool
- scar plastic or latex
- greasepaint (from palette or pencil – crimson lake, scarlet and brown)

Contracted scars

Paint *collodion* onto the skin and leave it to dry. Collodion causes the skin to pucker up and looks like a very old scar. The result is very subtle in appearance. It gives a good effect for contracted scars around a plastic scar and can also be used around burns.

Tip

A medical book is useful for reference. Cut out photos from the newspapers of accidents – these may be useful later as reference. Build up a varied collection to which you can refer necessary

Always test the skin for adverse reactions first, using a little where it won't show and not on the most delicate skin. If using collodion on the face, be careful not to place it too near the eyes.

Broken noses

Broken noses are created by lighting and shading the nose to look crooked. The skin must look inflamed and red. Wax can be used for any swelling, or sponge or cottonwool can be used, carefully, to plug the nostrils and so change the shape and create swelling.

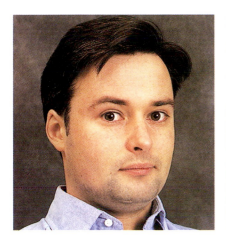

A broken nose
Before

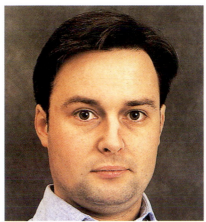

A broken nose effect has been created using shading and highlighting

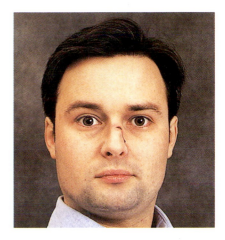

A small piece of wax has been added and cut into with a palette knife; 'blood' has been added

Activity – The 'beaten-up' look

This is a good exercise to practise on a male friend – usually it is male actors or stuntmen who have this type of make-up effect applied.

1 Place a piece of damp cottonwool in the mouth.

2 Model wax on either side of the nose, widening it at the top (to look swollen).

3 Place some cottonwool in the nostrils.

4 Using a rubber sponge, apply crimson lake greasepaint on top of a pale base across the forehead. Rub hard. Apply crimson around the left eye and on the chin and jaw.

5 Paint blue-grey under the left eye and on the lid and blend this into the red.

6 Use crimson lake pencil around the eyelids, close to the lashes. Blend it in.

7 On the same side as the red eye, highlight the bottom lip. Use cottonwool inside the mouth to make the lip protrude.

Equipment and materials

- cottonwool
- wax
- rubber sponge
- greasepaints (crimson lake, blue-grey, dark grey, burgundy and ivory)
- foundation (pale)
- pencil (crimson lake)
- toothbrush
- comb (small)
- coffee granules
- 'blood'
- water
- scar latex
- modelling tool or palette knife
- sealer
- isopropyl alcohol
- stipple sponge

8 Shade under the bottom lip with dark grey greasepaint.

9 Ruffle up the eyebrow. (Use a toothbrush or small comb to brush the eyebrows the wrong way.)

10 Smear coffee, 'blood' and water over parts of the left eyebrow and under the left eye.

11 Paint scar latex on the lower lip, or apply wax.

12 Using the flat edge of an artist's modelling tool or palette knife, cut into the material to lift the edge.

13 Add coffee and 'blood' mixture over the latex edge and a coffee granule on top.

14 Paint sealer over the waxed areas.

15 Clean the brush with isopropyl alcohol.

16 Paint grey greasepaint around the right eye.

17 Paint a burgundy bruise under it and on top of the eye, blending over the grey in parts.

18 Blend burgundy over the mouth area (above the cottonwool inside). Add burgundy to the left eye.

19 Place congealed 'blood' into the wax on the nose.

20 Using a crimson lake pencil or grease and a brush, make scratches on the forehead.

21 Put crimson lake on a stipple sponge. Scrape this over the cheeks and over the wax, to make stretches.

22 Add a running 'blood' and coffee mixture.

23 Blend ivory-coloured highlights onto the mouth swelling and a little on the nose.

Illness

1 Apply a pale foundation, very finely. If using panstik, apply it sparingly. Work it in so that it is not sitting on the surface of the skin.

2 Add a tiny amount of white foundation to the forehead, cheeks and chin. Work it in well.

3 Put a little blue and mauve greasepaint under the eyes (lines going down) and around the nostrils. Add brown shading in the corners of the eyes (as in ageing). Hollow out the temples and under the cheekbones.

4 Use dark grey-brown, sparingly, in circles under the eyes. Blend the edges. Put scarlet red greasepaint – toned down on the back of your hand – onto the eyelids. Place it close to the lashes and blend it upwards until it disappears. Do the same underneath the bottom lashes and add a little on the nostrils.

5 Use some high up on the cheekbones, unevenly, to look blotchy and feverish.

6 Place a little blue on the lips. Using a shading colour, emphasise the natural lines on the lips to make them look cracked. Frown lines can be added to denote stress.

7 Powder the make-up to set it.

Equipment and materials

- foundation (pale and white)
- greasepaint (blue, mauve brown, dark grey brown scarlet and blue)
- powder puff
- Vaseline
- glycerine and water in a spray bottle
- dropper

8 Smooth a little Vaseline on your fingertips and apply it lightly across the forehead and above the upper lip. Break the face up a little with shine, so that the light reflects on it.

9 To suggest perspiration, mix equal quantities of glycerine and water in a fine spray bottle. Spray it finely onto the forehead, where it will stick to the Vaseline. Dab the upper lip with water. (A dropper can be used for this – use a cleaned empty medicine bottle with a dropper.)

10 More red can be added to the eyelids and below the eyes, to close the eyelashes.

Illness: before and after make-up

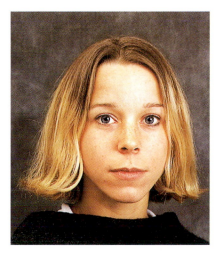 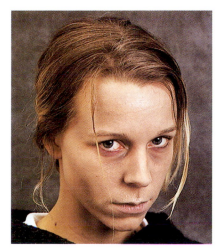

Equipment and materials

- greasepaints (purple, purplish black, maroon, yellow, crimson lake and black)
- fine brush
- powder puff
- fixative spray

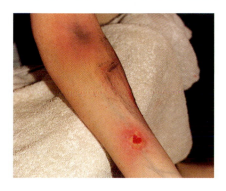

Drug addict

'Drug addict' effect

1 With your finger, dot purple greasepaint on either side of a vein on the inner wrist or arm. (Young girls tend to use veins around the ankles.)

2 Fade the purple to look lighter away from the vein.

3 Put a darker purplish black *along* the vein.

4 Using a maroon colour, make patchy areas around the veins.

5 Mix in yellow and blend this towards the outer edge. Don't do this uniformly: make it look raw and sore.

6 Using crimson lake, dot a few pinprick needle puncture marks.

7 Take a fine brush with black grease (or felt-tip pen) and put a *tiny* black dot on top of the red needle marks. Make some stronger than others.

8 Lightly powder or spray the effect with fixative spray.

'Drug addict' effect using collodion

1 Paint two coats of collodion.

2 Paint blue-grey grease irregularly on top of the collodion.

3 For added bruising, paint maroon, dark red or burgundy on top.

4 Powder, to set the greasepaint.

Equipment and materials

- collodion
- greasepaints (blue-grey, maroon, dark red and burgundy)
- powder puff
- sealer
- transparent nail varnish

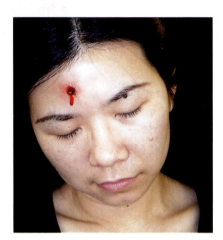

Bullet wound

Equipment and materials

- ballpoint pen (blue, black)
- colouring
- powder puff

Equipment and materials

- rubber stamp and blue inkpad
- felt-tip pens
- powder puff

Sealer or transparent nail varnish can be added to preserve the make-up for long shoots.

Bullet wounds

1   Paint red lipstick, or red greasepaint from your palette, onto the skin.
2   With an orange stick, apply a wound filler to the red, sore-looking patch, leaving different areas of light and shade.
3   Use a thicker, darker wound filler (add more black treacle to the mixture) and create different levels.
4   Put blushing gel or melted red gelatine on top.
5   Add running 'blood' to the wound.

Tattoos

Draw the design on paper first. Take into account whether it is a modern-day tattoo, or an old tattoo for a period film.

Temporary tattoos

1   For a one-day video shoot you can draw the tattoo freehand with a dark blue-black ballpoint pen, filling in the colours with coloured pencils or felt-tip pens. Alternatively you can transfer the design to the skin by drawing it first on tracing paper and then placing this on the skin, punching holes through the paper with the tip of your ballpoint pen to transfer the outline.
2   Fill in as usual with colour.
3   It is best to powder at the end when the design is dry: this gives a more natural-looking result.

Temporary tattoos can be bought in transfer form, but the designs are sometimes limited.

Longer term tattoos

1   For a tattoo effect that needs repairing every day over a long period of time, such as for a feature film or TV series, it is best to have a rubber stamp of your design made up to the correct size.
2   Use a blue inkpad to ink the stamp. Apply the stamp to clean, grease-free skin.
3   Colour in the tattoo with felt-tip pens. (Felt-tip pens provide a translucent stain which looks suitably long lasting.)
4   Finally, powder thoroughly when dry to take away the 'new' look.

Prosthetics

11

Introduction

Prosthetics are appliances made out of rubber, plastic, gelatine or any other material which can be affixed to the actor's face or body in order to change the shape. These three-dimensional pieces can range from simple effects, such as warts, scars or wounds, which do not require a lifecast, to more complex additions such as noses, chins, foreheads or eyebags which do require a lifecast – at least an impression of some part of the actor's face.

There are also the large mask-like creations of animals or aliens on blockbuster films in which whole head casts of the actors are taken and many people involved in the manufacturing process.

The effects (FX) industry has expanded and there are now companies across the world that take care of the whole process, from **lifecasting** to sculpting, moulding, running the foam, art working and application. Some companies will even fill the moulds that have been made by individual sculptors and return the prosthetics ready to be art worked and applied to the actors.

Some FX technicians team up with make-up artists who only apply, with one working in the lab and the other in the studio. In Britain the FX industry was pioneered by Stuart Freeborn who trained a lot of young people to help him create the original *Star Wars* movie characters. Many of his original assistants are now leaders in this field. In the USA Dick Smith led the way in developing techniques and training the following generations of technicians. Madame Tussauds, the museum of waxworks, is also to be thanked for training and employing its staff in casting, sculpting and making the moulds to produce their lifelike figures of famous people. Many have gone on to work in the film industry. There are niche specialities in this area as well, such as punching hair into the prosthetics to create hair styles, eyebrows and animal fur. Rather like wigmaking, it is important for the make-up artist to understand the entire process so that not only do they appreciate the work that goes into it, but can also recognise good quality when commissioning prosthetic pieces.

Good all-round make-up artists working in television and film will be able to create scars, noses, eye bags, swollen eye pieces, etc. out of gelatine. They will also have a high level of working experience in the art of applying and colouring them to blend in with the actor's face.

Tip

Ready-made prosthetics
Custom-made prosthetic pieces are available from professional make-up suppliers and are suitable for use in theatre and television for horror or fantasy effects. Such pieces are attached to the skin according to the manufacturer's instructions. Usually they are made of latex or plastic and fixed in position with spirit gum. The edges are sealed and blended with latex (eyelash adhesive is suitable) and the pieces are painted with greasepaint or camouflage make-up to blend in with the rest of the design.

How prosthetics are made

First a negative *lifecast* or *life mask* is made to match the actor's face or body part. From this, a *duplicate positive* casting is made with a material such as plaster or stone: this is called a *facecast* or *bodycast*.

Based on this cast, a new shape is sculpted (positive); from this a negative is made of the newly sculpted feature. A positive copy of the sculpture can now be made in a flexible material such as plastic, rubber or gelatine. This *prosthesis* or **appliance** is attached to the actor's face or body and coloured to blend in with the surrounding skin tone.

Materials used in casting and modelling

- **Plaster** This is the most basic ingredient and the cheapest. There are different types of **plaster**. *Plaster of Paris* is soft; *dental stone*, such as *Crystacal D* or *R*, is hard. Plaster moulds are usually reinforced with fibres or fabrics such as *scrim*, *sacking*, *hessian* or *horsehair*.
- **Clay** A good quality water-based clay is best. It must be kept wet and sealed inside a plastic bag. An oil-based sculpting material called **plastilene** can also be used. This has the advantage that it does not dry out, but the disadvantage that it does not give as smooth a finish as clay.
- **Alginate** This is used in taking accurate impressions of face or body parts. It takes about three minutes to set and can be accelerated by using warm water. (It is better to use

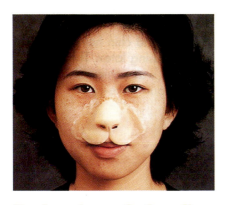

Ready-made prosthetics: a lion Before: the prosthetic piece is attached using spirit gum and latex is placed around the edges of the piece to blend away the hard edge

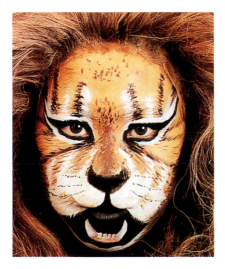

After: the lion make-up was produced using water-based make-up by copying a drawing of a lion

cold water to mix it, however, as the setting time may be speeded up in hot weather; alginate is affected by temperature.) It is pleasant smelling and harmless to the skin. It sets to a gelatine-like substance. Because this is floppy it loses its shape, so it must be backed with **plaster bandage** to reinforce the shape.

- **Gypsona** or **plaster bandage** This material is used in hospitals for setting broken bones. It is soaked briefly in water, wrung out and then smoothed over the alginate.

- **Silicone rubber** This is an expensive room-temperature vulcanising rubber compound, used for making flexible moulds. It must be used on large gelatine moulds and can be used on small moulds to give superior 'bite' to the mould halves. Silicone rubber work is usually done in specialist workshops as the material is expensive.

Materials used in making prosthetic pieces

- **Gelatine** A powder made from calves' hooves, used to make jelly. It is available as '300-grade technical gelatine'. It is mixed with glycerol and sorbitol and poured into hot moulds. When cool, it forms a rubbery compound. This is an easy and practical method you can use yourself.

- **Foam latex** This is a four- or five-part latex compound, which is whisked to a foam in a food mixer. The foam is poured into cold moulds and cooked in an oven to produce foam latex prosthetic pieces. These provide the best quality for large pieces and for close-up work for the screen. Foam latex work is usually done in specialist workshops as it is very time consuming and expensive.

- **Liquid latex** This is a milky liquid which can be painted as layers inside moulds to produce a solid rubber piece. Each painted-in layer should be applied thinly and allowed to dry before applying the next layer. This is easy to do yourself.

- **Plastic** In liquid form, as it is used for making bald caps, plastic also can be painted into moulds to make small prosthetic pieces. This also is easy to do.

Of all these materials, only two can be reused: gelatine, which can be heated, melted down and used again; **plastic**, which can be cut into small pieces and melted down in acetone.

Case Profile
Siobhan Harper-Ryan, Make-up artist

How long have you been in the industry?

I have been in and out of the film/TV industry since I was four but as a make-up artist for two years.

How did you get into it?

I felt it was a natural move for me. I had worked in front of the camera as a child, then as an adult I worked in costume. I have now found the career I am sticking with.

What or who has been your most significant project?

Each job has a significant point, but the job that allowed me to stretch myself creatively and challenge my organisational skills, was *Tales of Uplift and Moral Improvement*, Channel X for the BBC, 13 episodes, 200-year time span, special effects (FX) and Rik Mayall as an elderly lady.

What do you enjoy most about your work?

Being creative. Transforming an actor in the make-up seat. Researching for period productions and characters. Realising the director's dream and meeting lots of great people.

And least?

Night shoots in December! Doing my accounts!

What advice would you give to people trying to get into this area of work now?

Show willing. Experiment in your spare time. Keep contacts you make on set. Be calm in the make-up room and on set. Be willing to work for no payment when starting out. Most of all, find a course which suits you and work hard. You will be rewarded.

Flat plate moulds

Flat plate moulds are among the most useful moulds. All moulding techniques can be considered as embellishments of this basic technique. It is ideal for making wounds, scars, stitched wounds, keloid scars, blisters, burns and so on. These can be made in advance and kept until you need them.

This type of mould-making can be done on any worktop or kitchen table and does not require a lifecast of the actor's facial features.

Making the mould (negative)

Making the flat plate

1   Take a plastic box about 50 mm deep. Half-fill it (to about 25 mm) with dental stone plaster to create the flat plate. You will be sculpting on top of this plaster, so make it smooth on top. (Scrim can be added into the mix for reinforcement.)

2   When set, take the plaster slab out of the box and cut three *keys* in the sides (off-centre), using a small saw. These will allow you to check later that the mould halves are correctly fitted together.

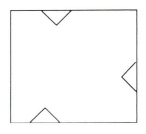

**Flat plate moulds –
Three keys are cut into the
sides of the plaster slab**

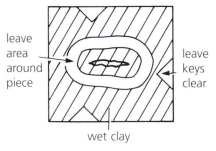

leave
area
around
piece

leave
keys
clear

wet clay

Casting

Equipment and materials

- plastic box (about 50 mm deep)
- dental stone plaster and scrim
- small saw (for cutting the keys)
- shellac (to seal the mould)
- Vaseline
- sculpting tools
- clay
- screwdriver (to separate the moulds)

3 Coat the flat plate with *shellac* and Vaseline, to seal the plaster. If you do not have time for this, use Vaseline only. (Clay put onto dry plaster will shrivel up.)

4 When dry, it is ready for sculpting on.

Sculpting

Sculpt your piece using wet clay – scars, wounds, bumps and flaps of skin are all suitable for flat plate moulds. Leave plenty of room around the piece. Blend away the edges, using a damp sponge or brush.

Casting

1 Make a low wall in wet clay around the piece, leaving 6–12 mm of clear plaster around the edge of the piece. *Do not cover the keys*.

2 Apply Vaseline all over the exposed plaster – the keys and the areas around the piece.

3 Place the whole plate inside the box. Press the clay walls to seal against the edge of the box walls.

4 Mix another batch of plaster and fill the box to the brim, reinforcing with scrim. Take care that the plaster has filled the details of your sculpted piece.

5 Allow the plaster to set, which will take about 40 minutes. As it sets, the plaster will first get hot and then become cold.

Removing the mould

1 Take the completed mould out of the box. Separate the two halves carefully, using a screwdriver to lever if necessary.

2 Clean all traces of wet clay from the mould.

3 Put both halves in the oven to dry (just over 100°C) for at least two hours.

4 When dry, shellac both halves of the mould (inside). The moulds are now ready for filling with gelatine.

The separator

A separating material, sometimes referred to as a *parting agent* or *releasing compound*, is used to help moulds detach easily when they are pulled apart. It is also used to seal the moulds, to prevent moisture from penetrating the surface. Vaseline (or petroleum jelly) is the most commonly used separator. Another separator is a saturated solution of soap and water, which is used when casting with foam latex.

Equipment and materials

- 100 g fine powdered gelatine
- 200 g liquid sorbitol
- 200 g glycine (glycerol)
- $\frac{1}{2}$ tablespoon of zinc oxide powder
- scraped pancake colour

Filling the moulds with gelatine

Using gelatine

Mould gelatine, as in the following recipe, *must never be used directly onto a person's skin*. It would cause burns. It must be used only for filling moulds.

1 Mix the liquid sorbitol and glycerine with the gelatine. Heat moderately, until the mixture has clarified. It will still contain many bubbles.
2 Mix together in a small bowl zinc oxide and pancake scrapings – 6W to 10W pancakes, depending on the required skin tone – with a little gelatine, until you are happy with the colour. Add this to the heated mixture.

Ideally, this mixture should be made up in advance to allow time for the bubbles to rise and disperse. It can be kept indefinitely (cold) in a plastic bag or container and reheated when needed.

Variations

- Less gelatine makes a softer, weaker appliance; more gelatine makes a harder, tougher one.
- To make a clear gelatine for blisters and the like, leave out the zinc oxide.

Colouring

- Any powdered *pigment* can be added to create a colour. It should be combined with glycerine in a separate bowl before being added to the mixture.
- Liquid *food colouring*, mixed with a little *isopropyl alcohol*, can also be used.
- *Chopped crepe hair* can be added to produce a vein texture.

Preparing the mould

The mould must be hot, but not too hot.

1 Place the mould in a moderately heated oven for 15 minutes.
2 Remove the mould from the oven and wipe the inside with Vaseline.

Filling the mould

1 Pour the hot gelatine mixture into the mould, making sure that the piece is well covered and there are no air bubbles.
2 Close the mould halves, matching the keys to one another. Apply pressure evenly – do not press hard and then release or air will be sucked back into the mould. Put a stage weight or similar on top of the mould and leave it for about two hours, until cold. (Do not try to open a warm mould: the gelatine inside will be a sticky mess.)

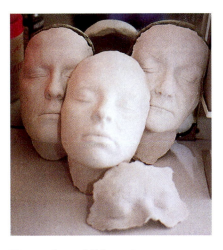

Examples of lifecasts

Opening the mould

1   Separate the mould gently, using powder to stop the edges rolling over and a modelling tool to lift the piece. Care is needed here if you are to achieve the best possible piece.

2   When the piece is free, pull off the excess edges around the piece. It is tempting to leave them on, because they will be beautifully thin, but the best edges for application are close to the piece itself.

What went wrong?

If the edges are really thick, there are only four possible causes:

1   The mould did not close properly. Check it against the light for any trapped pieces of plaster or similar obstacles.

2   The gelatine was too cool. Try again, with warmer gelatine.

3   The mould was too cool when the gelatine was poured. Warm the mould.

4   Not enough pressure was applied during the cooling period. Add more weight.

Lifecasting from the actor's face

Caring for the actor

Many people – not just actors – are nervous of having their faces covered in plaster in order to provide a lifecast. This is quite understandable, and care should be taken in discussing the person's particular anxieties before the casting session. You should experience a lifecast yourself before undertaking one on another person. Students should practise on one another to help them understand why lifecasting is sometimes frightening for actors. When lifecasting in a film studio, it is usual to have the unit nurse present during the procedure. In a classroom, a nurse or teacher with a knowledge of first aid procedures should be in attendance, in case of emergency and to provide a reassuring presence.

For actors, lifecasting sessions are similar to visiting a dentist. The procedure is out of their control, leaving them vulnerable and helpless. Take time to explain how they will breathe under the cast. Actors must be reassured that if they wish, at any time and for whatever reason, the lifecast will be removed immediately if they simply raise an arm in a pre-arranged signal. The sympathetic, calm manner required of a make-up artist in all her work is of prime importance when lifecasting.

Equipment and materials

- one large plastic cape
- one bald cap
- alginate
- plaster bandage (pre-cut in 150 mm and 300 mm strips)
- scissors
- petroleum jelly or silicone grease to cover facial hair (including eyebrows and eyelashes)
- mixing bowls
- spatulas
- brushes
- water
- plaster
- permanent marker
- salt
- tissues and cotton wool
- towels

Taking the lifecast (negative)

All tools and materials must be laid out in preparation before the appointed time. The equipment must be neatly arranged and ready to hand. Measure the required amount of alginate powder into the bowl. Make sure there are enough strips of plaster bandage in different sizes: you will need enough to cover the face with three or four layers.

Preparing the actor

1   Seat the actor comfortably and wrap the plastic cape around him. He should be wearing comfortable clothing – roll-necked sweaters are not suitable as the plaster may drip onto the neck. Use towels and tissues tucked into the neckline to protect clothing and to keep the actor warm.

2   Position the bald cap over his head to protect his hair, making sure that it covers the hairline.

3   Apply Vaseline, KY jelly or any silicone grease to the eyebrows and eyelashes in a thin coating. Do the same with any other facial hair, such as a beard or moustache. (Alternatively, these can be plastered down with wax, but remember to apply grease on top of the wax so that the alginate does not stick to it.)

It is important to talk to the actor while preparing him for the lifecasting. Make clear to him that if he signals you to remove the alginate from his face, you will remove it from the nose, the mouth and the eyes, in that order. This should help to relieve the claustrophobic feeling he may be undergoing. Explain to him that the alginate will feel very cold at first but will warm up later.

Applying the alginate impression material

Whilst the **alginate** is being applied the actor should remain as still as possible and in an upright position. The face must not be tilted in any direction, either up or down or from side to side; otherwise the impression will not be accurate.

1   Having prepared the actor, start mixing the alginate by adding cold water to the powder. Stir from side to side to avoid trapping air in the mix.

2   When the mixture is a creamy paste, apply it to the face, beginning on the forehead and working down over the face. Leave the nose and mouth until last. *Remember to leave breathing holes around the nostrils*. Use a brush to apply the alginate in particular areas. This will ensure that no air bubbles are trapped under the alginate. These areas, known as the undercuts, are beneath the chin and jawline, the mouth, the eyes and around the nostrils. (Instead of using a brush you can run your fingers gently along these points.) Keep the actor's nostrils clear. If there is a blockage, ask him to expel air sharply through his nose to shift it. An airway should also be allowed through the mouth.

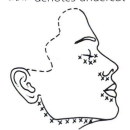

✗✗✗ denotes undercut

Taking a lifecast

Reinforcing the alginate with plaster bandage

3   When the alginate has been applied smoothly, dip the wads of pre-cut plaster bandages into warm, lightly salted water. Squeeze out excess water before applying the plaster bandage to the alginate. (For extra support, a layer of rough towelling can be placed over the wet alginate before applying the bandage. This should not be necessary if you use plenty of plaster bandage.)

4   The alginate will have set – setting takes approximately three minutes – and you can now begin placing strips of plaster bandage over the life cast. Keep inside the edge of the alginate: *plaster bandage should not directly touch the skin* as the alkali in the plaster can cause irritation.

5   Having covered the face with four layers of the bandage all over the alginate, you may add an extra strip around the outside of the bandaged area to provide additional support when removing the cast. Keep an eye on the actor, talking reassuringly and watching for the agreed hand signal.

6   When you think the plaster bandages have set, run your fingers around the edge. About ten minutes is usually sufficient for the plaster to harden.

Removing the lifecast

Ask the actor to wriggle his face gently under the lifecast in order to loosen the alginate. He should lean forward, holding the cast in his hands. As he moves his facial muscles, the cast will loosen and fall into his hands. Alternatively, you can lift the edges of the lifecast, making sure you are lifting the alginate and not just the plaster bandage, and work the lifecast loose.

Taking care of the actor and the lifecast

As soon as the lifecast has been removed, the actor's face must be restored to normal.

1   Remove any pieces of plaster and alginate from the face with damp cottonwool. The actor can now wash his face with warm water and soap.

2   After drying with a clean towel, an astringent may be used to close the pores of the skin; rosewater is excellent for this purpose. Finally, a mild moisturiser should be gently applied.

3   Insert plugs of wet clay, wax or plastilene into the nostrils of the cast, so that the liquid plaster will not leak. Position the cast gently on a bed of towels, ensuring that the nose does not get damaged. Alternatively, while you mix the plaster, ask a helper to cradle the cast in his or her lap, supporting the mould with cupped hands.

Making a positive plaster cast

Preparing the plaster cast

Mixing the plaster

1   Put two or three cups of water into a bowl, then slowly sift the plaster into the water until it barely rests on top of the water. Always mix plaster into cold water. Let the mixture stand until it begins to thicken. The plaster will draw up the water and become fully saturated: this process is called *slaking*.

2   Begin mixing with a side-to-side motion, then bang the worktop surface next to or underneath the bowl to bring any trapped air to the surface. Gently blow on any bubbles to disperse them. The consistency of the plaster should be like pouring cream.

Filling the mould

3   The shell, or mould, is ready to be filled with plaster. When the plaster has been mixed thoroughly, begin by painting some of it into the mould, using a soft brush. Brush the wash of plaster into all the cavities.

4   Pour the plaster into the mould, building it up slowly as the plaster thickens. *Pour from one end only*. When the plaster has thickened to a trowelling consistency, begin to apply it with increasing thickness to build up strength in the lifecast. There should be at least 25–50 mm thickness throughout the mould. Do not overfill or the cast will be too heavy to handle. Leave it for one hour.

5   When hardened, pick it up and turn it over. Remove the plaster bandage and alginate from the inner mould, taking care not to damage the face impression. Finish the cast by filing away any rough parts, and if necessary scratch the name of the artiste on the underside of the cast.

6   Leave the cast to harden and dry out overnight.

Finishing the plaster cast

Give the cast a coat of shellac to seal the plaster. The shape of the feature you wish to reproduce will be modelled in clay onto the facecast.

Sculpting the new feature

Sculpting is the most important part of prosthetic work. The piece, however skilfully cast and whichever material it is in – plastic, gelatine, liquid latex or foam latex – will only be as good as the shape you have created in clay. Whatever your concept, the skill of modelling and sculpting the piece requires much practice.

Modelling the feature

- a sketch and/or Polaroid photographs of the required shape
- various modelling tools, in wood or metal
- bowl of water
- spray bottle filled with water
- clay or plastilene
- rough towel, grapefruit peel or coarse stipple sponge

1   Place your facecast on a work surface, supported underneath by some lumps of modelling clay or plastilene to hold it in position. Place a small amount of wet clay onto the part of the face that you wish to change, often the nose.

2   When you have achieved the shape that you want, begin to put in the details. Keep the clay damp by spraying it with water; clay that is too dry does not produce good results. Remember to sculpt very thin edges, using your wet fingers to smooth away the base of the feature until it blends into the surrounding area of the facecast.

3   Take into account the final texture of the modelled feature. It should blend with the surrounding skin in the area to which it will be applied. Texture can be added by gently pressing a rough-textured towel or piece of grapefruit peel onto the clay surface. Alternatively, a coarse-textured stipple sponge will have the same effect.

Activity – Sculpting a face

Using wet modelling clay, sculpt a life-sized face using a photograph or a sketch for reference. Try to achieve a good likeness. Build up the shape of the face using small lumps of clay, a bit at a time. Remember to keep the clay damp by spraying it with water every few hours. When you are not working on the face, wrap it in plastic to prevent it from drying out.

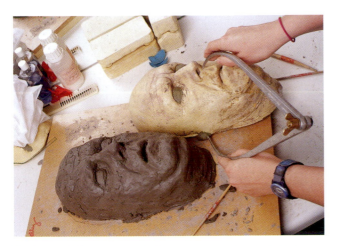

Using callipers to obtain exact measurements

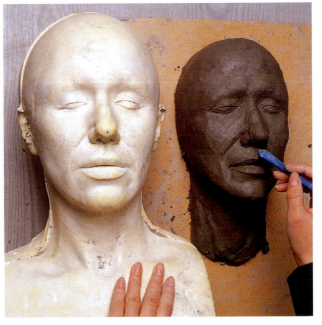

Sculpting a face in clay using a plaster cast for reference

Casting the mould

1 To cast the newly modelled feature into a mould from which you can make your prosthetic piece, it is necessary to build a wall around the feature. Modelling clay or plastilene can be used for this. The wall should be even in height and higher than the newly modelled nose (or other facial feature).

2 Using your fingertips, spread a thin layer of Vaseline on the nose and the surrounding area lying inside the clay wall.

3 Mix plaster as before, but less will be needed. Paint on a thin coat of plaster using a brush, then pour plaster to cover the nose. Bang on the table with your fist to disperse air bubbles in the plaster. Leave it to dry.

4 When the plaster is dry, remove the clay wall and separate the nose mould from the remodelled lifecast.

5 Remove the modelled nose from the interior of the mould and smooth away any imperfections with a file.

Cleaning the mould

Wash the mould in warm water, using a clean soft brush in all the cavities. Leave it to dry overnight, when it will be ready to fill with the chosen material.

Making the prosthetic piece

The prosthetic piece can be made out of plastic, latex or gelatine. There are three latex techniques: *painting in*, *slush*, and *foam*. The foam latex method will be explained at the end of the chapter.

The painting method

The new nose shape can be made by painting the inside of the mould with successive layers of liquid latex. Prior to application, the latex can be coloured by mixing in scrapings of pancake or food colouring to give it a flesh tone or other effect, as desired. When the latex is dry it will be darker in colour.

1 Before applying the latex, brush the mould with liquid soap.

2 Pour a little latex into the mould and use a brush to paint the inside of the mould until it is covered. Allow each layer to dry before painting the next.

3 Paint the next layer beyond the edge of the piece.

4 Apply about 15 layers, so that the piece will hold its shape. Concentrate the most latex on the middle part of the piece, so that the edges are thin.

5 Leave the casting for six hours, during which it will become darker in colour.

The slush method

The slush method uses latex, but without painting it in layers. As with the painting method, the area inside the mould should be brushed with liquid soap, which will act as a release agent.

1 Pour the latex into the mould and sluice it around, tilting it gently so that the latex runs into the required places.
2 Build up thickness in the middle, but leave the edges thin.
3 Leave the cast overnight to dry.

Colouring the latex

The liquid latex is milky white and can be coloured by adding scrapings of pancake or food colouring to give it a flesh tone or other effect, as desired. Remember that when the latex is dry, the colour will be darker.

Using plastic

Equipment and materials

● Vaseline
● plastic
● pancake

This method involves using liquid bald cap plastic and painting layers into the mould. Again, the positive mould is not used.

1 Spread a layer of Vaseline inside the mould (as a release agent).
2 Paint in layers of plastic, allowing each layer to dry before painting in the next. Scrapings of pancake colour and the like can be mixed into colour the transparent plastic.
3 As with the latex nose, more layers should be concentrated in the middle part of the nose mould and the edges left thin.

Case Profile
Stuart Sewell, Prosthetic special effects artist

How long have you been working in the industry?
Ten years.

How did you get into it?
I had an interest in films from quite a young age. Attending a local art college (in Stourbridge), I began to develop my draughtsman and sculpture skills. This coincided with my first beginning to lifecast faces and sculpt simple masks. After this GAD in art and design, I applied successfully to Bournemouth and Poole College of Art and Design. I worked my way through a two-year HND course in film and television. This allowed me to understand how films are made in general.

What or who has been your most significant project?

For me, *Lost in Space*: it was the first time I ran a department. Having a good crew around me made this happen. That was very exciting – people like Andy Hunt, Connor O'Sullivan, Susan Howard and Dan Nixon. It's fun when the crew gels, perhaps even the best part.

What do you most enjoy about your work?
Sculpting and problem solving, especially creating a one-off make-up effect.

And least?
Ludicrously tight schedules and politics.

What advice would you give to people trying to get into this area of work now?
Have a thick skin.

Equipment and materials

- talcum powder
- soft brush
- powder

Removing the prosthetic piece from the mould

Caring for the prosthesis

1   Use talcum powder and a soft brush to lift and peel the edges carefully, powdering with the brush as you go. This prevents the material from sticking to itself as you remove it.

2   When you have removed the prosthesis from the mould, powder it inside and out with more powder. This is to remove any grease from the Vaseline, if the prosthesis is plastic, or soap if it is latex. Keep the prosthetic nose in its mould to retain its shape until you are ready to use it.

Caring for the mould

The mould should be washed in soap and water and allowed to dry naturally. You can make as many pieces as you like from the mould and it will probably be necessary to produce several before you get a good result.

Do not be disappointed if your prosthetic pieces do not turn out as well as you hoped. This happens all the time to experienced prosthetic specialists.

The facecast can be used for experiments in making all sorts of pieces: eyebags and jowls for ageing; a forehead for a monster make-up; a clown's nose; a witch's nose and chin – the possibilities are endless. Each piece must be modelled and a mould made of each feature in the same way as you did for your first nose. To make a mask you can remodel the entire facecast with clay and cast it to produce a full face mask.

Sectional lifecasting

When only a section of the face is needed – often the nose – instead of taking an impression of the whole face you can lifecast just the feature itself. This is less time consuming and is also cheaper than casting the entire face.

Taking a cast of the nose

1   About half of the eye sockets and cheeks should be covered, as well as the nose itself, to allow sufficient room for good edges on the final positive.

2   The eyebrows, eyelashes and any moustache should be coated with Vaseline to protect them and to allow ease of separation. The person's nostrils can be plugged with cottonwool covered with Vaseline, as he or she can breathe through the mouth.

3   The alginate and the plaster bandage are applied in the same way as for the previous facecast, using smaller quantities of

Equipment and materials

- Vaseline
- cottonwool
- alginate
- plaster bandage
- dental stone

plaster. Allow a few minutes for the plaster bandage to harden before removing the cast from the face. Ensure that the artiste's skin is restored to its normal state.

4 When the cast (*negative*) has been removed from the face it can be used as a mould. Pour in the freshly mixed plaster (dental stone – Crystacal D or R) and leave it to set.

5 When the plaster has hardened, remove the new plaster cast (*positive*) from the mould. Correct any minor defects, trim and smooth the surfaces.

Making a gelatine nose

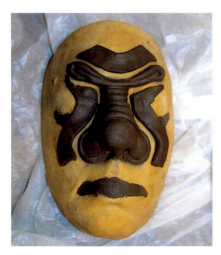

Nose modelled on face cast ready for coating in plaster

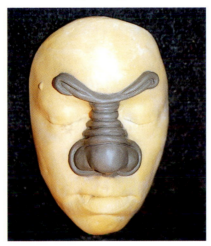

Gelatine nose ready for application to the face

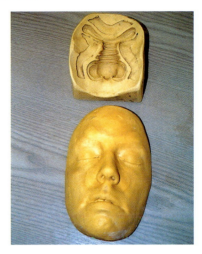

Nose cast separated from face cast and gelatine nose removed

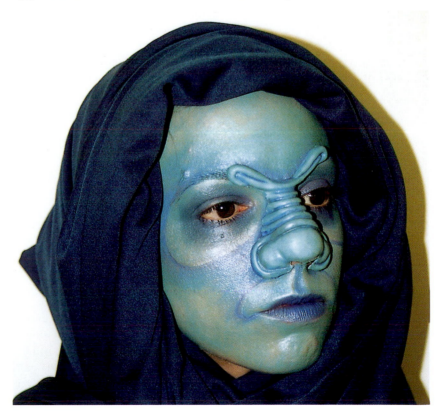

Final effect: the gelatine nose applied to the face and make-up added to create an alien look

Sectional casting

Making the plaster block for the nose

For **sectional lifecastings** it is neater to *box* the features in a rectangle, making a block for the nose. The walls can be made of clay, metal, lead or damp-proof plastic.

Making the positive mould

1   Make a watertight wall around the feature, with a 12 mm gap all round.
2   Mix a batch of thick plaster (dental stone Crystacal D or R), and pour a base for the lifecast section.
3   Once the base is thick enough to support the lifecast feature without it sinking into the freshly mixed plaster, lay the lifecast on top of the base. Pour the plaster around the feature to set it in the block.
4   When the plaster is hard, remove the walls. Smooth out any lumps by sanding or scraping the plaster slab and feature.
5   Cut three keys in the sides, off-centre.
6   Apply Vaseline to the feature.

Sculpting the prosthesis

1   Sculpt the appliance, using wax, clay or plastilene on top of the stone feature. Blend the edges down and away from the feature so that the edges will be thin.
2   Sculpt an overspill or trench with clay around the sculpture, about 6–12 mm thick and 6 mm away from the edge of the sculpture. This creates an overflow, for use if you later want to use foam latex or gelatine to make the prosthetic piece. This overflow or trench is called the **flash**.

Making the plaster mould (negative)

This stage consists in building the other half of the mould:

1   Build a box wall in the same way as you did for the positive half. The wall should be high enough to reach 20 mm above the feature.
2   Using a sponge or brush, blend the outer edge of the flash to the walls to seal the edges and to make the box walls watertight.

To cast the mould, use Crystacal plaster, a little thinner than you did for the positive half of the mould.

3   Mix some plaster and water – always add the plaster to the water and not the other way round – and pour it slowly *around* the modelled piece (not onto it). Blow on the plaster and keep pouring until the piece is covered and the box mould filled. Tap the underside of the workbench to bring any air bubbles to the surface. Leave the plaster negative to set in its box.

Equipment and materials

- sponge or brush
- plaster (Crystacal)
- screwdriver or chisel

4 When the plaster has set, remove the walls and trim the plaster.

5 Leave for two hours, then gently prise the mould apart. (You may need a large screwdriver or chisel to help.)

Cleaning the mould

Wash the mould in warm water, using a soft brush in all the cavities. Leave it to dry overnight, when it will be ready to fill with the chosen material.

Gelatine prosthetic pieces

Equipment and materials

- Vaseline
- gelatine
- powder
- modelling tool
- plastic bag

Gelatine is good to work with because it is reusable. If the piece is not as successful as you would have liked, you can melt it and try again.

Filling the mould

1 Seal the mould with Vaseline.

2 Heat the gelatine (using the same recipe and method as for the flat plate moulds) and heat the moulds in an oven until hot.

3 Sluice a little of the gelatine around the mould to pick up the surface detail, then pour in more gelatine to fill the mould.

4 Close the mould and leave for two hours or until cold.

Opening the mould

Gently separate the parts of the mould and remove the gelatine piece from the positive mould. First powder it and use a modelling tool to lift it. Then powder it further, to stop the edges rolling over as you peel the prosthesis out of the negative mould.

Storing gelatine pieces

Keep all gelatine pieces in an airtight plastic bag.

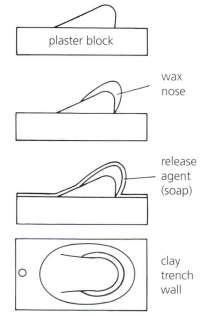

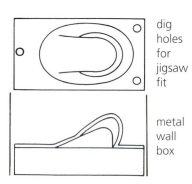

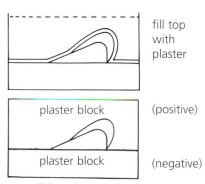

Making the plaster block for a foam latex or gelatine nose

Applying a prosthetic piece

The adhesives

Various adhesives are available, which have different uses in applying prosthetics:

- **Spirit gum** will stick latex, gelatine and plastic.
- **Dow Corning 355 medical adhesive** will stick latex, plastic and gelatine – instantly. It can be thinned for easier application and for economy, using Tipp-Ex thinner or trichlorotrifluoroethane.
- **ProsAide** will stick latex pieces only, but when mixed with water it can be used as a sealer on foam pieces. When mixed with a thickener (Cabosil), it can also be used as a paste to conceal the edges of a piece. When mixed with artists' acrylic paints, it can be used to artwork the piece. This should be done in advance, before application.
- **Duo** will stick latex and blend the edges of latex prosthetic pieces.

Sealing and preparation

1   Seal the prosthetic piece with sealer. Allow it to dry.
2   Prepare the piece for fixing, removing any unwanted edge material.

Affixing the piece

Equipment and materials

- sealer
- powder
- adhesive
- cloth or powder puff
- modelling tool or spatula

1   Position the prosthetic piece on the actor's face and powder around it to show the outline.
2   Remove the piece and put a thin layer of adhesive on the underside of the piece, in the middle. Do not apply adhesive yet to the edges of the piece.
3   Position the piece carefully and press it with a cloth or powder puff.
4   Stick the edges last, using a modelling tool or small spatula to hold up the edges and to prevent them from curling or sticking together.

Blending the edges of the piece

- If the piece is *gelatine*, use **witch hazel** on a cotton bud to blend the edges. Use the dry end of the cotton bud to press firmly and roll on the edge.
- If the piece is *latex*, use Duo on a modelling tool to seal the edge onto the skin. Smooth the Duo with a palette knife. Alternatively, you can use ProsAide mixed with Cabosil to a paste to blend the edges.

- If the piece is *plastic*, use a cotton bud with a small dab of acetone to blend the edges of the piece. *Do not touch the skin*, only the edge of the piece.

Colouring the piece

Once the piece has been fixed and sealed you can paint it. Some make-up bases are made especially for prosthetic work. Camouflage make-up is excellent for coverage and for matching the skin tone of the surrounding skin area. Use rubber stippling sponges to achieve a dappled effect and build up the textured effect using several colours. Powder between layers. Be careful not to overdo the colouring. You cannot wipe away unwanted make-up from a prosthetic piece. When painting prosthetic cuts and wounds, put colour into the cut early: the bright colour will draw the eye to it and thereby distract attention from the edge.

When applying make-up to the piece, remember that the prosthesis will appear lighter than the skin – use a darker tone than on the rest of the skin, therefore. Warm pink tones should be stippled on the piece before the skin tone colour, exactly as when working with wax.

Take extra care when working near the eyes. *All adhesives are potentially dangerous*. Avoid any prosthetic work involving the eye areas until you are experienced. Even then, undertake such work only with extreme caution.

Removing the prosthetic piece

Pieces attached with spirit gum

1   Use a small brush dipped in mild mastix remover to remove the prosthetic piece. Apply the remover to the edges around the piece. Lift it with one hand, as with the other you work the brush to loosen it.

2   Clean the spirit gum from the actor's face with cottonwool dampened with the mastix remover.

3   Remove the make-up in the normal way.

Pieces attached with Dow Corning 355

Use a keratin-based oil called Klene-All. Isopropyl alcohol also dissolves the adhesive.

Pieces attached with latex

Use warm water and cotton buds.

Foam latex pieces used to transform a young woman into an old man

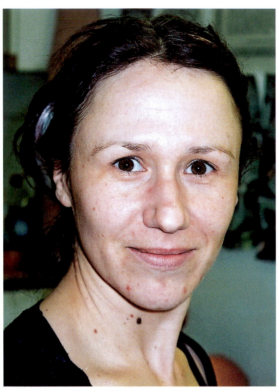

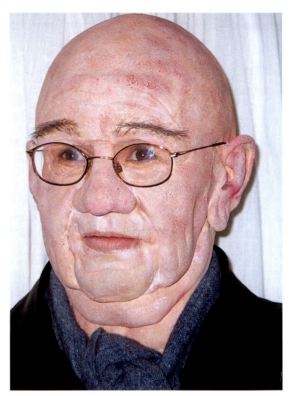

Before   After

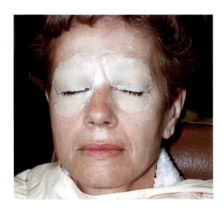
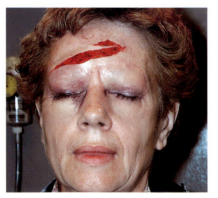
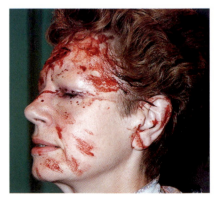

Gelatine pieces used for a casualty effect by Christine Powers for TV series *Casualty*

A patient arriving at casualty from a simulated train crash. To achieve the look her face was cast and two eyes and one forehead pieces made from gelatine to enable the make-up artist to do swellings and cuts. The pieces were then applied, using spirit gum and blending the edges with witch hazel. The pieces were then made up as skin. Casualty effects were applied on top to create the gruesome effect.

The need for care

Great care should be taken when removing prosthetic pieces. Your understanding of the types of adhesives must include knowledge of the materials needed to remove them. As more products become available in the field of make-up there is greater choice, but with increased choice comes increased responsibility.

Some adhesives are not suitable for use around the eyes, but can safely be used on the chin or nose. This is not because of danger from the adhesive, which should always be safe for use on the skin, but because of danger from the product used to *remove* the adhesive.

Allowing time

In cases where there is substantial use of prosthetics, as with fantasy or 'cartoon' character make-up, you need to allow as long to remove them as to apply them. It is understandable if actors feel like tearing the pieces off, but it is crucial that you do not let this happen. Although patience and understanding are always essential parts of the make-up artist's job, they are absolutely vital when applying and removing prosthetics.

 Activity – Producing a face mask

1 Take an impression of a fellow student's face.
2 From this impression, make a positive cast.
3 Model new features onto the positive cast, for example, to make a monster's or a witch's face.
4 Make a negative mould of the new face.
5 Use the slush latex technique to produce the face mask.

Using latex: foam technique

Developments in technology

The advances in technology have affected the prosthetics laboratories and workshops more than any other area of make-up artistry. The technology advances all the time developing new methods and new materials. To appreciate the time and effort involved and to excel in this area, try to do some work experience or apprentice yourself to a professional prosthetics workshop and learn the art and technology of this remarkable aspect of make-up. The specialist makers of prosthetics are part chemist, part artist and part engineer. Each tends to specialise in a particular area, such as sculpting, mould making, foaming latex, knotting hair into the pieces, colouring or artworking. A complicated ageing sequence or character change as it is eventually seen in a film may have used many prosthetic pieces and relied on the work of an entire crew of talented people.

Commissioning foam latex pieces

Large prosthetic pieces need to be made out of foam latex as this is the lightest material and most similar to natural skin. Most make-up artists will commission a specialist to make the pieces for the production. In these circumstances, you will be required to take the actor to the prosthetic specialist's workshop for a lifecasting session. Several visits may be necessary to ensure the quality and fit of the prosthetic piece or pieces required. Here are some aspects to look out for:

1 Make sure that the piece fits exactly when the actor's face is mobile.
2 Check that the edges of the piece are so fine and thin that they blend into the surrounding skin.
3 Check that there are no large air bubbles in the piece.

Don't be afraid to put forward your own ideas to the specialist. You will be the one applying the prosthetics in the studio and by that stage it will be too late to correct any faults. If you have a difference of opinion with the specialist, however, don't talk about this in front of the actor. Sort out any problems when he or she isn't there. If the actor thinks that anything is wrong, she or he will lose confidence.

When the foam latex pieces arrive from the specialist workshop, they should have been washed in soap and water to remove the strong smell of chemicals and dried carefully. This is important, as the smell can be unpleasant and distracting for the person wearing the piece. The number of duplicate pieces will be whatever you have ordered. With foam latex you need a new piece on each day on the shoot.

Tip

The ingredients for making foam latex can be purchased in small batches and mixed according to the maker's instructions. They are usually named 'Parts A, B and C' by the manufacturers.

Making foam latex pieces

Foam latex

The best but most expensive method of casting is to fill the mould with foam latex and cure it in an oven. This approach requires much more preparation and time than any other type of prosthetic work. It is undoubtedly the finest method available for three-dimensional effects for the media. For large pieces in particular the foam latex surpasses all other methods; it is light and flexible and adheres well to the skin. If the film or TV budget can afford foam latex pieces, it is advisable to contract the work out to an expert. Many make-up artists have neither the desire nor the skill to work in this area, but every make-up artist should have some knowledge of the techniques involved in making foam latex appliances.

Foam latex has the following ingredients:

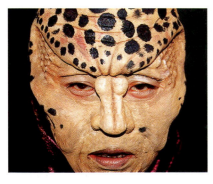

Foam latex pieces used for an alien fantasy look

Tip

Colour can be mixed into the gelling agent, using artist's tube colours thinned with water. For example, flesh colour can be obtain by mixing a teaspoon of burnt sienna with a quarter teaspoon of water.

- **Latex base** A high-quality chemically thickened latex, sterilised with ammonia.
- **Foam agent** An emulsion of soaps: when whisked with the latex base, these produce a foam.
- **Cure agent** A mixture of sulphur and other chemicals that *vulcanises* the foam latex when it is *cured* in the oven.
- **Gel agent** An acid that turns the latex from a liquid to a semi-solid: it coagulates the foam, preventing it from breaking down. Warning: *Before it has been cured, this is highly toxic.*
- **Soap release**   The release agent which is painted onto the plaster moulds before filling them with foam latex. This ensures that the foam can be removed easily without sticking after the casting has come out of the oven.

The prosthetics room

The prosthetics room should be equipped with an electric food mixer and bowl, weighing scales, a drill and a prosthetics oven for curing the moulds. (Warning: *An industrial mask should be worn as some of ingredients used in mixing foam latex are known to be toxic.*) Inhaling plaster dust is bad for the health, so it is safest to assume that most of the work in the room is detrimental to one's health and a surgical or dentist's mask should always be worn. For large effects, using full heads and bodies, catering mixers and ovens are used.

The temperature and humidity of the workroom affects the foaming process: higher temperatures cause faster setting, lower temperatures make it slower. It is not practical to attempt foaming operations at below 15°C (60°F). For professional results, you need air conditioning and heating. All other aspects of making prosthetic pieces can be carried out quite successfully in college, at home in the kitchen or in a garden shed – but it's not so simple for foam latex mixing and curing. Here chemistry and make-up overlap; successful results rely on dedication and experience.

Health and safety

The foam latex technician works with highly toxic and dangerous ingredients. (Warning: *It is dangerous to inhale the products.*) To minimise the risks of accidents, follow these rules:

1   Keep all chemicals out of reach of children and inquisitive adults.
2   Do not decant chemicals into other bottles, especially bottles which have been used for drinks. To do so is an unnecessary risk and could prove fatal if someone mistook the chemical for a drink.
3   Always wear a respirator and goggles when opening bottles that are old or newly purchased. The vapours and fumes can build up to dangerous levels inside the containers.

4   Never sniff or breathe in any of the chemicals used in making foam latex.

5   Always put the lids back on the bottles, making sure that they are tightly sealed.

6   Wash any accidental splashes of chemicals from the skin with cold water immediately.

7   Keep eyewash solution and an eyebath near the sink in case of accident.

8   Never leave a mess in the workshop. Always wipe worktops with disinfectant and wipe machinery immediately after use. Wash used moulds. If the work area is clean, tidy and organised, it will also be safer.

9   The workshop should be spacious and well ventilated. Extractor fans should be used near open windows to get rid of the vapours from the ammonia present in the latex.

10 Wash your hands before and after working with foam latex.

11 Always read the labels on the bottles, especially the labels warning of risks. Always read the instruction sheets included with the products and take heed of the health and safety warnings.

12 Wear goggles and gloves; if working in a poorly ventilated workshop, wear a respirator approved for ammonia vapour.

13 Never drink or eat in the foam lab or workshop. Food and drink can become contaminated with chemical vapours.

Tip

Small quantities of the ingredients for foam latex can be weighed in plastic cups which can be thrown away after use.

When measuring out the gelling agent, it is helpful to use a spoon that has been waxed: this prevents the gelling agent from sticking to the spoon.

Equipment

The actual process of making the foam latex is very simple but, rather like making a soufflé, it can go wrong without one understanding why. As with cooking anything, variations in the mixture or the cooking times can upset the balance. When the foam fails to rise or has too many air bubbles, it is usually necessary to start all over again.

Filling the moulds and curing the latex

Preparation

1   Apply soap release to the plaster moulds and allow this to dry.

2   Weigh out the ingredients in plastic cups.

Mixing (foaming the latex)

3   Add the latex base, foam agent and cure agent to the mixing bowl.

4   Turn on the food mixer at *high* speed for 3–6 minutes, depending on the rise wanted; the greater rise (volume), the softer the foam.

Equipment and materials

- the moulds you wish to fill
- soap release
- soft brush (to apply the soap release)
- food mixer with a large bowl
- plastic cups (for measuring the ingredients)
- accurate weighing scales
- spatula
- stopwatch (to time the process)
- electric oven (to bake the moulds)
- latex base (150 g)
- foam agent (30–45 g)
- cure agent (17 g)
- gel agent (4–10 g)

5 Turn down the mixer to *medium* speed, to refine the foam and break down the bubbles, for 4 minutes.

6 Turn the mixer down to a *slow* speed to refine the foam even more, for a minimum of 4 minutes.

7 Add the gel agent slowly and mix it into the foam. Mix the two together for at least one minute.

8 Stop the mixer and fill the moulds carefully. Make sure that no air is trapped under the foam.

9 Close the moulds together.

10 Leave the foam until it gels. To test for gelling, with fingertips press the overspill of foam at the side of the mould.

Curing

11 Place the foam-filled moulds into a pre-heated oven at 100°C (212°F). Bake them for 3–4 hours until the foam inside the moulds has been cured.

12 Remove the moulds from the oven, and allow them to cool down before opening them. Test the texture of the foam by pushing a spatula into it: it should be springy and sponge-like. When fully cured, it will spring back to its shape.

13 Wash the pieces in soapy water, then dry and powder them.

Foam lab technicians usually keep a *log* of their foam runs. This helps them to compare temperatures and cooking times with the quality of the results. An accurate record provides continuity and encourages improvements in foam latex work.

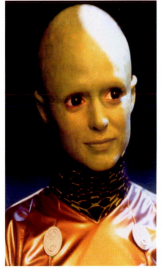

Prosthetic ears and foam latex bald cap on Heather Graham for *Alien Love Triangle.* Prosthetic supervisors Conor O'Sullivan with Stuart Sewell

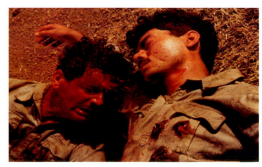

Chest wounds for *Captain Corelli's Mandolin.* Prosthetic supervisors Conor O'Sullivan with Jo Allen

Ganesh God project by Siobhan Harper Ryan

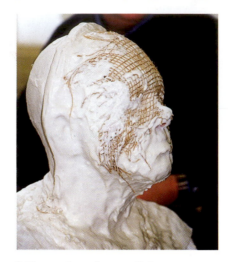

Lifecasting the model

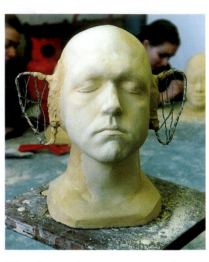

Wire is used to create ear shape

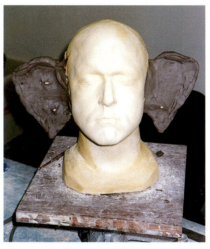

Clay is added and sculpting begins

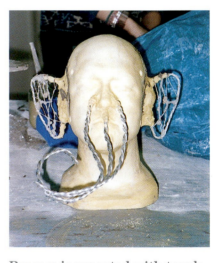

Process is repeated with trunk

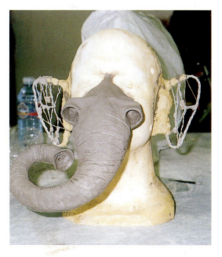

Sculpting the trunk

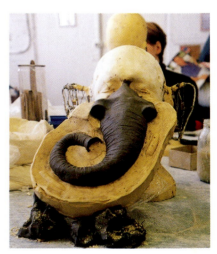

Moulds are taken of all sculpted pieces

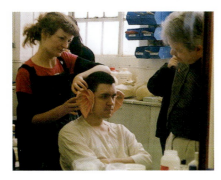

Positioning the pieces

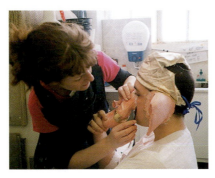

Foam latex pieces are secured in place

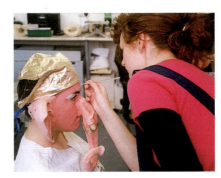

Finishing touches are added

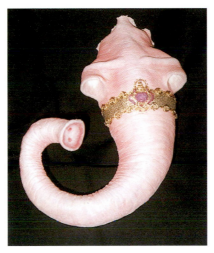

The finished trunk

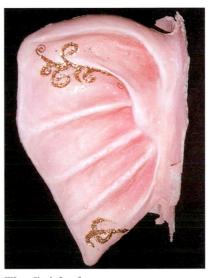

The finished ear

The finished project

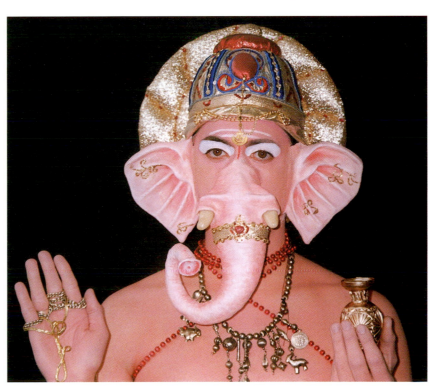

Case Profile
Conor O'Sullivan, Prosthetics supervisor

How long have you been working in the industry?
Eleven years.

How did you get into it?
After getting a degree in marine biology, I followed my interest in sculpting which I have always had (my mother was a sculptress) and joined a company as a SPFX runner.

What or who has been your most significant project?
The Hours (2001), directed by Stephen Daldry and starring Nicole Kidman and Julianne Moore. I made and applied a nose on Nicole Kidman and did a prosthetic ageing on Julianne Moore, partnered by Jo Allen.

What do you enjoy most about your work?
Characterisation, technical and artistic problem-solving people and working with the people involved in the business.

And least?
Sometimes having to work with people who combine over-ambition with little talent.

What advice would you give people trying to get into this area of work now?
Be prepared for the long hours, be persistent but not irritating, and above all be patient.

Casualty effects on *Saving Private Ryan*. Prosthetic artists Conor O'Sullivan and Stuart Sewell

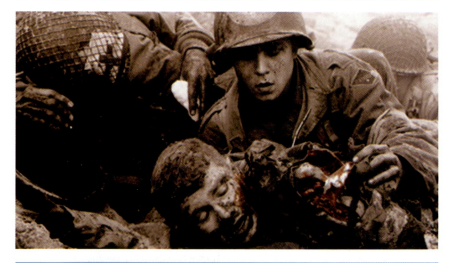

Activity – Making a prosthetic nose

1 Take an impression of the subject's nose, using alginate compound and plaster bandage.

2 From the impression, make a positive cast.

3 Model the required nose shape onto the positive cast.

4 Make a negative mould from the modelled nose.

5 Separate the mould from the model.

6 Fill the mould with latex foam. Push the *positive* lifecast into the *negative* mould. Cook in a pre-heated oven at 100°C (212°F), or according to the manufacturer's instructions.

Character make-up

12

Introduction

A fine character make-up, like a fine painting or performance, is the result of thorough preparation, intelligent selection and skilled execution. Through the script and rehearsals, the actor becomes acquainted with the physical appearance, background, environment, personality and age of the person he or she is portraying. As make-up artists, it is our job to translate this information into visual terms.

Sex change

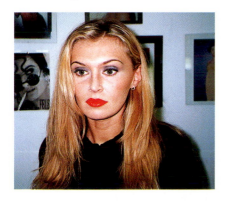

Before

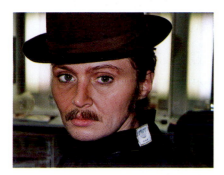

After

Often the actor and the director will have very firm ideas on how the particular character should look; the make-up artist must interpret their ideas. The script may specify the character's health, occupation and personal attributes. The make-up artist, through the make-up, should help the actor to interpret the role and add credibility to her or his performance. If a man is supposed to be returning from a long stint in the West Indies, for example, it would look wrong for him to be pale in colour; similarly, a suntan would look ridiculous on a woman of high birth in Victorian times, because such women never exposed their faces to the sun. Each character should be analysed thoroughly in this way and the make-up tried out until everyone is satisfied with the result. Physical appearance is determined by factors such as these:

- heredity
- race
- environment
- temperament
- health
- age

Though these factors are not of equal importance when analysing a character, they constitute a useful checklist when carrying out your preparation and research.

Planning the make-up

Every technique of media make-up is drawn on in creating a character make-up, yet the make-up should be limited to what is really necessary for the result to be convincing. Character make-up may therefore entail merely adding a moustache and a subtle ageing effect. Alternatively you may need the whole works: wig, facial hair, false nose, strong ageing effect, and so on. Whatever the production demands, it is up to the make-up artist to work out the best way to achieve it. The type of production will impose practical constraints:

- whether it is for television, a feature film, a video, the theatre or a commercial shoot
- how much the budget allows for materials and the costs of specialist suppliers
- how long is allowed for the make-up artist to achieve the result

In character work there are three categories:

- people in fashion
- people no longer in fashion
- people ahead of fashion

Pay attention to the recorded evidence concerning when it was fashionable to have facial hair, for example, or when women wore heavy make-up. Remember, though, that there are always people who are not at all influenced by fashion: men who have beards and moustaches when others don't and women who wear no make-up when others do. In period films, the make-up artist should try to recreate normal people and not always what was in fashion. When creating a character there are five important factors to consider:

1   Age.
2   Temperament.
3   Social standing.
4   Race.
5   Period.

Bearing these factors in mind, here are some general guidelines in approaching character make-up:

- If you don't need it, don't use it.
- If you do use it, know why you're using it.
- Try to draw out the character through the use of make-up.
- Don't work on artistes – work with them.
- Don't stick rigidly to the rules – instead, draw on all the techniques you know to obtain the maximum effect.
- For character make-up, mix many different colours and stipple them to give great depth and life to the face.

Tip

Design the make-up on paper first. Spend time on planning and organising your selection of materials and resources.

Activity

Choose one of the following subjects and create a character make-up for a colleague or model:

1 *A witch* – using make-up, a false nose and chin (with prosthetic pieces): suitable for a stage performance.
2 *An elderly Victorian man* – using make-up and including facial hair on lace or directly applied loose hair: suitable for a feature film.
3 *A geisha girl* – using make-up and including oriental eyepieces made with plastic or latex: suitable for a photograph.
4 *Changing a woman into an Indian man* – using make-up and including beard stubble: suitable for TV.

Case Profile
Julia Wilson, Make-up artist

How long have you been in the industry?
Since 1984 – 17 years.

How did you get into it?
I had done an art foundation course and beauty therapy course and by chance they needed artistic people to apply prosthetic ears on all the local Africans on *Out of Africa* and to do 1930s–1940s crowd make-up.

What or who has been your most significant project?
Several: *Out of Africa* because it made me realise what a fun/creative rewarding job it is so I went into more training courses; *Tomb-Raider*, travelling to Cambodia, exquisite temples and monks; a TV series called *Shackleton*, living off an icebreaking boat in the Arctic, working as a complete team in and out of each other's pockets and space, getting on and off 'icebergs' in Arctic equipment, on and off dinghies knowing that if you fell into the icy water you have four minutes to live, using only 'Reel colour' palettes for weathering and burnt faces because normal water-based foundations would freeze on the face!

What do you enjoy most about your work?
The travel – meeting different people, experiencing different cultures in countries – the closeness and bonding between actors and units. The challenges that one has to face, for example, certain prosthetics or body painting. The creativity! Above all, how rewarding it feels if you have completed your job well and the rest of the crew compliment your work and the actor is happy and confident in you.

And least?
The long hours and driving to and from locations, especially after period make-ups where you have to set and dress wigs and facial hair, etc. after work. It can make it a 16- or 18-hour day!

What advice would you give to people trying to get into this area of work now?
Always be enthusiastic and keen to learn and practise a lot at every opportunity. Be prepared to work long hours. It is exhausting sometimes. Try and get on a job on a film or in TV as a trainee and watch and learn from other people, always working hard with initiative and without an attitude. You would hopefully then get taken onto other jobs where you meet more people and networking starts. Don't be disheartened – it's a long ladder.

Contact lenses

It is not always necessary to use prosthetics and wigs to achieve a dramatic change in an actor. In feature films, **contact lenses** are sometimes used for dramatic specific effects – white contact lenses can make the eyes look blind, for instance; red ones can make them look horrific.

This type of effect is very expensive: the lenses must be made specially for the actor. An assistant make-up artist is needed, to look after the lenses, to clean them and to stand by the actor at all times to check that he or she wears them only for the time allowed and in case of problems such as dust particles. The optician will advise on how long the actor should wear the lenses each day and the make-up artist should observe these instructions for the actor's safety. This kind of effect is out of the question unless the production can afford the necessary time and money.

Young and old Make-up artist Tom Smith

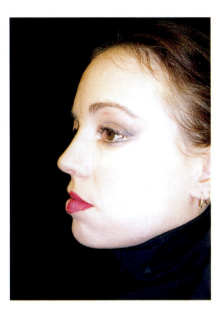 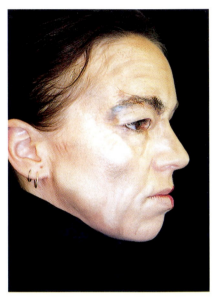

Directly applied hair on eyebrows and prosthetic eye pieces and make-up

Look-alikes

In recreating a well-known person, the make-up artist aims to achieve as accurate a likeness as possible. The actor will generally be cast with the likeness in mind, but even so there are often adjustments to be made.

Begin by comparing the face of the character and the artiste. Analyse the differences and similarities. Examine the skin tones, shape of the face, colour of the eyes and hair and shape of the eyebrows and nose.

When the character is relatively modern – such as Marilyn Monroe or Marlene Dietrich – there will be numerous photographs available for use as reference and details of the person will be widely known. For instance, it is common knowledge that Marilyn Monroe never

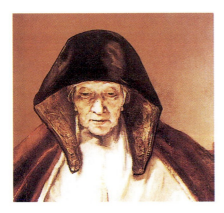

Look-alikes: a Rembrandt painting

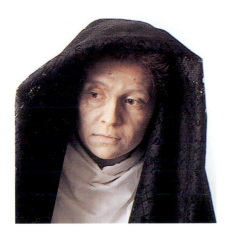

A model made up to look like the painting

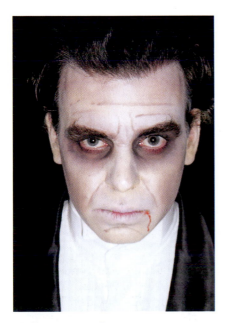

Halloween make-up

sunbathed, even though it was fashionable to do so. As well as having the famous blonde hair and arched eyebrows, the **look-alike** would need to have a pale skin. Similarly, if the subject were Abraham Lincoln it might be necessary to model a nose for the actor in order to achieve a likeness. Points of similarity should be emphasised and differences minimised.

In the case of famous people from history who predate photography, such as Elizabeth I, we have to rely on portraits or caricatures. Very often the painting or engraving will have simplified the personal features. Go back further still into history and there is only the information handed down through historical records. The tombs of Tutankhamen, for example, provide evidence of the fashions in make-up and hair in ancient Egypt. Many people think of Cleopatra in terms of how Elizabeth Taylor looked in her film role opposite Richard Burton as Anthony, but in fact these portrayals had 1960s overtones reflecting the period in which they were filmed.

When a portrait or engraving is the only evidence of how the person looked, bear in mind that the artist has used brushmarks or cross-hatchings to represent shading or lighting. As the make-up artist, however, you must create a realistic effect with subtler shading and lighting. You may also be required to adapt the look somewhat for present-day audiences. Thus, a very long beard for a medieval period production might be disallowed by the director on the grounds that it would seem too bizarre, even though an existing portrait of Edward II of England shows that he actually had such a beard. A film accurately based on eighteenth-century life would look unbelievable to us. We may know from records that the ladies at court wore thick layers of white lead on their faces, but it would look extraordinary to our eyes. The make-up artist would therefore use pale skin tones, but would avoid the overpainted look that was in fact accepted in those days.

Some historical figures who are household names, such as Winston Churchill, J.F. Kennedy or Charlie Chaplin, are within living memory and so well known that they must look right when played by actors. There is an abundance of photographs and archive material to help the make-up artist achieve the likeness, but it is then particularly important that the actors should be physically similar to the characters they are to portray, so that they can easily be transformed by the make-up artist. Make-up and hair must be carefully researched and planned in such cases. With the help of photographs from books and old newspaper cuttings, make notes and sketches. Photographs of the actor will be useful so that you can compare the two faces and plan what you will need to do for the make-up and hair.

You will need to experiment on the actor's face and maybe change your design accordingly. Adapting the make-up to the face requires that you study it from every angle. Whereas a photograph or painting is frozen for all time at one angle, the actor must move and be seen in three dimensions and may need to be filmed in bright sunshine and in dimly lit interiors.

Character make-up is as important in characterisation as the clothes and the lines. If the likeness has been recreated skilfully, the actor will be able to perform the role with much greater effectiveness.

Boxer
Make-up artist
Siobhan Harper-Ryan

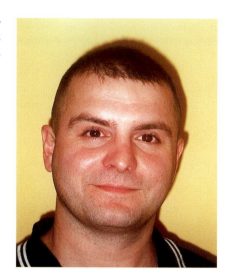

Before

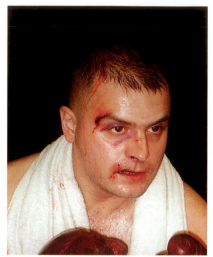

After

Ethnic appearances

Equipment and materials

- greasepaints
- powder
- brushes

Caucasian to oriental

It is possible to give a subject an oriental appearance simply with make-up, using highlights and shadows.

Chinese eyes using make-up

1 Highlight the entire eyelid and add shading at the inner corners and underneath the outer corners.

2 The effect can be improved by plaiting the hair on either side of the temples and by pulling to lift the skin.

Tom Smith doing a character make-up on a student using eye pieces

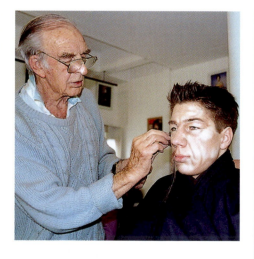

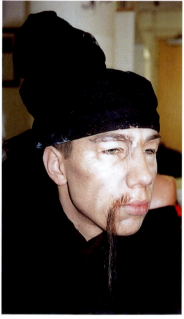

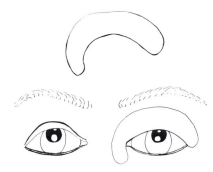

Oriental eyes: the eyepiece, and the eyepiece in place

Equipment and materials

- eyepieces
- spirit gum
- make-up

Equipment and materials

- wax
- towel
- cotton buds
- eyeliner (brown)
- greasepaints (dark brown, Chinese yellow, yellow and green)
- powder and brush
- stipple sponge (rubber)
- tissues
- eyeshadow (navy blue)
- pancake (black and dark brown)

Chinese eyes using eyepieces

A more realistic look can be obtained by using plastic eyepieces. The eyepieces are made by painting PVC and PVA into a *negative* mould taken from modelled oriental eyes.

To place them in position:

1 The actor must be sitting upright and looking straight ahead, with both eyes open.

2 Dab the eyepiece with spirit gum.

3 Place the eyepiece above the actor's eye on the inner (nose) side. Draw it across the eyelid so that the lower edge is covering the lid, allowing the lid to open and close freely.

4 Stick the false eyepiece at the outer corner of the eye.

5 Apply make-up to match the rest of the facial make-up.

Caucasian to Indian

For a female

1 To change the nose shape, apply wax; press with a towel, to give texture to the wax. When modelling around the nostrils, put a cotton bud in the nostril and model around this. Seal the wax.

2 Use a brown eyeliner on the inner eyelid to give an almond shape.

3 Apply a dark brown grease as a base.

4 Go back to the nose, adding another coat of sealer; powder when dry.

5 Add Chinese yellow and dark brown to colour the nose.

6 Apply eyeliner on the upper lid and smudge this.

7 Add more dark base on top of the nose, coming down the nose in patches (use a rubber stipple sponge).

8 Place yellow highlights over this – on the forehead and on top of the mouth, to break up the skin texture; also above the cheekbones and in the inner corners of the eyes, blending into the dark colour. Do the same under the eyes.

9 Put some dark brown on the lips, lightly and unevenly.

10 Put dark brown down the side of the nose. Blot with a tissue and powder.

11 Put brown shadow over the eyelids and a tiny amount of matt navy blue shadow under the eyes.

12 Draw the upper eyelines with dark brown and black pancake.

13 Fill in the eyebrows, with dark brown drawn underneath; extend this to the ends of the brows.

14 Darken the skin a little more if necessary, with dark brown and green.

The main points to remember are these:

- the dusky stain around the eyes and the lips
- taking the redness out of the skin
- the colour – yellow, to counteract the red
- the curve of the nose characteristic of Indian people.

For a male

When making up a Caucasian man as an Indian, use pencils and grease (dark brown) to draw in lines, as in ageing make-up, and apply hair to make and dress a moustache. The method of make-up is this:

1   Apply the base in patches, not all over.

2   Put dark brown on the forehead (two sections above the eyebrows).

3   Stipple burgundy on the cheeks, the beardline and the chin. Blot with a tissue.

4   Stipple green greasepaint onto the beardline to put it back. Use a little red also.

5   Use Dermablend to cover any spots or shadows under the eyes.

6   Add grey or brown grease on the upper lids.

7   Paint grey eyeliner underneath, to break up the texture and remove the 'made-up' look.

8   Pencil grey on the eyebrows if needed – just one or two strokes.

9   Stipple dark brown onto the forehead.

Suntans

Applying a suntan

Ask the actor what colour he normally turns in the sun. Remember that some areas, such as the forehead and the cheeks, may go browner than others.

1   Stipple crimson lake panstik on those areas.

2   Go over the top with a yellow-brown colour to avoid the colour looking too pink.

Applying sunburn

1   Stipple red on the areas mentioned above.

2   Ask the actor to crinkle up his eyes: pat over the resulting wrinkles at the outer corners of the eyes.

3   Do not powder the make-up: leave it to shine.

Fantasy make-up

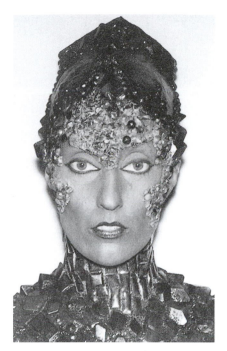

Fantasy make-up for *Dr Who*

Fantasy make-up is fun to do and satisfies the creative side in every make-up artist. The effect can be the simple painting of an animal face, a witch or a clown, or the design of more complex monsters using prosthetics and bald caps. Fantasy can be beautiful and charming, or dramatic and frightening.

Any materials may be used in order to achieve the desired fantasy effect, but in general it is advisable to use *grease-based products* (such as panstiks) for the stage, as watercolours tend to run when the actor gets hot. For photographic, TV and film work, watercolours for the face provide excellent results, with strong, clear colours.

Ready-made prosthetic pieces such as latex noses or ears are ideal in creating fantasy characters such as animals. By cutting a few pieces from a broom or sweeping brush, whiskers can be stuck onto the animal face for the finishing touch.

When making up dancers for light entertainment shows, the brief often given is to create a bold, striking effect. Shiny eyeshadows, glitter and strong colours may be used to blend with the costumes and scenery.

Of all the areas of make-up, fantasy is the one which offers the make-up artist the greatest freedom of expression. Occasionally when working in films there will be a scene such as a carnival, when everyone is in fancy-dress costumes and fantasy make-up is required. Give your creativity and imagination free rein!

Bald caps

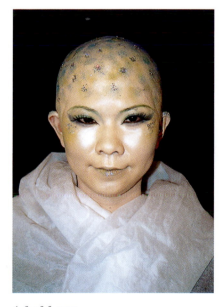

A bald cap

The purpose of a bald cap is to cover some or all of the actor's hair so that the person looks bald-headed. In television and film work, this is often a key factor in making a character look older.

The cap needs to be strong enough to hold its shape, yet fine enough to be invisible – especially at the edges, which must be matched into the surrounding skin tones. Bald caps in the theatre are usually quite thick. They have to be put on and taken off many times and in any case they are seen from a distance. Similarly, bald caps used in clown make-up are not intended to be realistic. Traditionally these are made of thick rubber, like a bathing cap, with brightly coloured synthetic hair sewn into or stuck onto them. In film and TV work, however, the material must be fine enough to look realistic even in close-up.

In ageing make-up the bald cap will often be worn with a toupee over the top, so as to show a bald patch or a receding hairline. In fantasy make-up the artist can instead use the bald cap as the basis of colourful designs.

Bald caps are easy to make, though time consuming. Ready-made caps can be bought from professional make-up shops, ranging from the inexpensive thick ones to the more expensive types made of fine quality plastic which can be stretched to fit any size of head.

Step-by-step fantasy bald cap

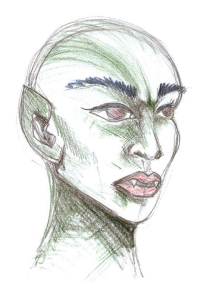

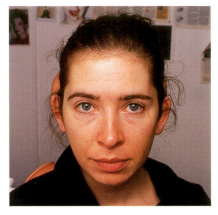

1 Model Catherine Hawkes before make-up.

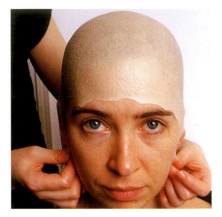

2 Pre-made plastic bald cap is pulled over on head, attached with spirit gum and blended to skin gently with acetone.

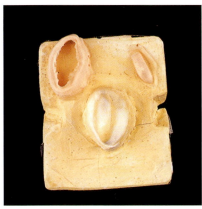

3 Pre-made sculpted foam latex ears.

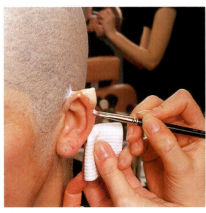

4 Foam latex ears are stuck down in place with Prosaide using a small brush.

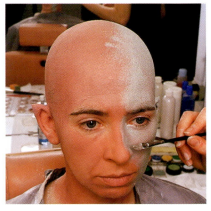

5 Green creme make-up is applied by stippling colour with latex sponge.

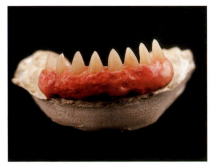

6 Teeth have been pre-made from a cast of model's own teeth.

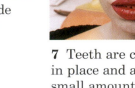

7 Teeth are carefully inserted in place and attached with a small amount of Polygrip.

Make-up artist Siobhan Harper Ryan

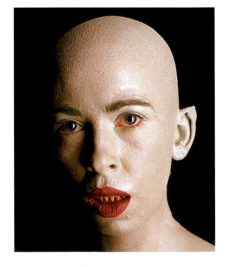

8 Finished look.

Making a bald cap

Equipment and materials

- clingfilm
- clear adhesive tape
- eyeline pencil or a crayon
- dressmaker's tape measure
- head block

Making a template

The method used in taking a pattern for a bald cap is similar to that used in taking a pattern for a wig.

Stage 1: Making the pattern

1. Tie back the hair. If the model has long hair, pull the ponytail band down lower, and add more clingfilm at the base. You need at the end to have a clingfilm head shape, reinforced all over with overlapping layers of adhesive tape.
2. Lay clingfilm across the head.
3. Ask the artiste to pull the clingfilm down, making sure that the sideburns are covered.
4. Place one long strip of adhesive tape around the head. The actor can now let go of the clingfilm.
5. Slowly go round the whole head with adhesive tape, slightly overlapping it. When cutting lengths of tape, do so away from the actor – the noise can be irritating. Do not pull the adhesive tape too tightly on the head.
6. Go around the hairline with a crayon or eyebrow pencil. Draw in the ears as well. Cover the pencilled lines with adhesive tape, to protect them from being rubbed off.

Stage 2: Taking measurements

1. Using a dressmaker's tape measure, measure above the ears round to the bone at the fullest part of the back of the head. This is the circumference of the head.
2. Measure from the front hairline to the nape of the neck.
3. Measure from temple to temple.
4. Write these measurements and the person's name on the cap. Again, cover the writing with clear adhesive tape.
5. Draw a horizontal line across the front, to show the pattern's position when straight. When the cap is put on the block you will then be able to check that it is again straight.
6. Cut the pattern upwards to the top of the front of the ear, so that you can take it off the actor's head. Place your hands on top of the pattern to lift it off.
7. Cut around the hairline that you have drawn. Allow a 12 mm margin in addition, as the plastic will shrink.

Stage 3: Transferring the pattern to the block

1. Turn the moulded head pattern inside out.
2. Place the pattern onto the **head block**. Check that it is straight and central.

3   Holding the pattern firmly with one hand, draw a line around the hairline, at least 12 mm away from it. Go under the ear and down the back, marking the line on the head block.

4   You now have the pattern drawn on the head block and you can put the pattern aside.

Note: Sometimes the head block you are using will be either too small or too large for your pattern. Adjust by allowing more or less width.

Plastic caps

Bald cap plastic comes in liquid form, comprising *PVC* and *PVA* plus a *plasticiser*. A number of the formulations in use combine *acetone*, as a solvent, with a plasticiser to give elasticity to the product. Cap plastic can be tinted with any colour of your choice: you can add scrapings of pancake, powdered food colouring, raw pigments, or face powder.

The fumes of the solvents are very strong. It is essential that the work be carried out in a well-ventilated room, with open windows and an electric fan to blow the fumes out of the windows. Alternatively, if the weather permits, the work can be carried out in the open air.

The cap is made by painting layers of the plastic onto a solid head block. Unless you are using a metal block, you must first spread Vaseline on the block. Most people use plastic head blocks as these are lighter.

Each layer of plastic will take about ten minutes to dry. Do not apply the next coat until the previous one is dry.

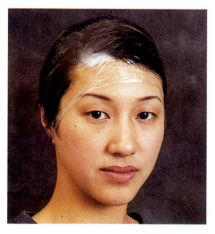
Wrapping clingfilm around the head to make the head pattern

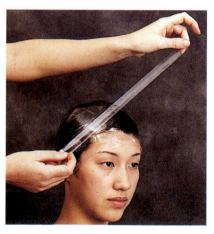
Sticking adhesive tape over the top of the clingfilm to secure the head shape

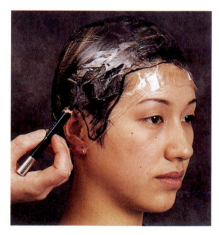
Drawing the hairline and the ears

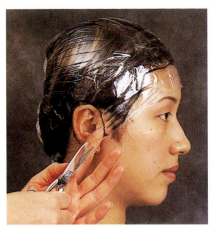

Cutting a small slit in the middle of the drawn ear shape in order to remove the pattern

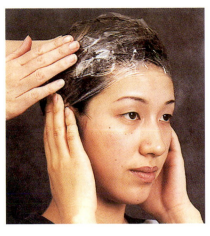

Removing the pattern from the head

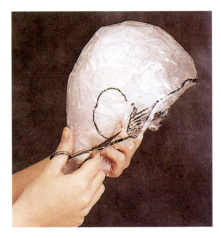

Cutting around the hairline

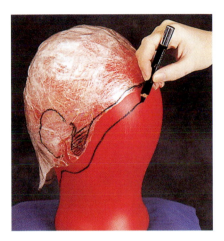

The head shape is placed on the block and a line is drawn approximately 12 mm beyond the hairline

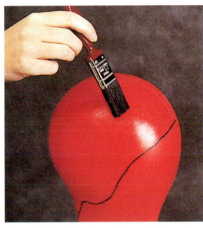

Vaseline has been applied, and now cap plastic layers are being applied

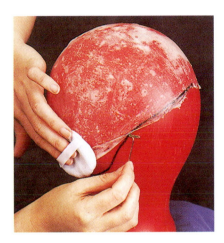

Removing the bald cap from the block with a T-pin and powdering

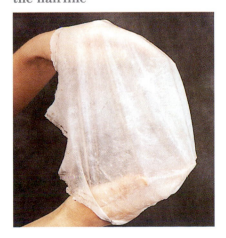

The stretched bald cap

Applying the cap plastic to the block

1   If there are any grooves in the centre join, file them down and smooth them out with mortician's wax.

2   Prepare the head block by smearing over it a very thin coat of Vaseline, which should then be wiped over with a tissue.

3   Apply the liquid plastic using a large brush – a small house-painting brush is suitable. Have to hand a jar of acetone, so that you can clean the brush after each layer. (You will need about three layers all over the cap and to the edges; and a further three, with colour, in the middle. Extra layers can be applied to the back to give more strength in attaching the cap to the head.) Apply the first layer of plastic thinly and quickly. Be methodical and don't reapply plastic over the same area. Work from the top to the edges, keeping them as thin as possible.

4 Leave the layer to dry. You will be able to tell when it is dry because of the change in colour of the plastic. Clean your brush with acetone.

5 Apply two more layers, each time working slightly inside the outer edges so as to give the finest edge possible. Keep to your method, applying the plastic quickly using gentle strokes. Avoid air bubbles and don't allow any hairs or clogged plastic to come off the brush. While waiting for layers to dry, keep your brush in acetone to prevent the hairs from sticking together.

Colouring the plastic

1 For the final three layers of plastic you will usually want to add some colour. Add a blob of your base colour – whatever is required, from natural to green – to the plastic and stir it well until it has been thoroughly mixed together. You can use prosthetic paints, ground-up pancake, or powder pigments.

2 Apply the final three layers to the top and back only. Each layer should finish slightly further from the edge than the previous layer, as with the earlier applications.

3 To reinforce the back, apply further layers or place very fine hair lace between the layers of plastic. Leave a small amount of lace free of the edge of the cap. This is what you will use to stick the cap to the skin.

4 When this third or final layer of plastic has been applied, leave the cap to dry thoroughly, preferably overnight.

Taking the bald cap off the block

1 Brush the edges of the plastic with talcum powder. Without tearing the plastic, carefully slip the T-pin between the cap and the block. Gently release the edge all the way around, powdering the inside as you go.

2 Ease the cap free a little further in, again with the pin and the powder.

3 Once you have enough to hold securely, pull the cap from back to front.

4 When the cap is free from the block, powder both sides. Put it back onto the block, inside out, until required for use.

Rubber bald caps

Though most bald caps nowadays are made of plastic, they can be made using latex rubber instead. The method then is to stipple the latex onto the block using a sponge.

To test a bald cap, stretch it out: on release it should return to its original shape quickly. Look also for unwanted air bubbles.

Refronting a plastic cap

- hair gel
- scissors
- acetone
- Duo
- cotton buds
- tissues
- spirit gum or surgiccal adhesive
- powder puff
- wooden modelling tool
- stipple sponge
- make-up

Old caps can often be reused, but you then need first to put a new edge around, the hairline. This process is called refronting. There are two sides to a cap made of plastic: the top side is shiny, the underneath is matt.

1 Put a tiny amount of Vaseline on the surface of the plastic head and powder it with talcum or face powder.

2 Put the cap onto the plastic head, pulling the edges out.

3 Using acetone, gently wipe the edges underneath. This sticks the cap down and dissolves the edges. (Acetone is a solvent for bald cap plastic.)

4 Pour cap plastic into a jar.

5 Scrape some pancake of the appropriate colour onto a tissue and sprinkle the scrapings onto the cap plastic.

6 Pour a little into a dish. Using a brush 50–75 mm wide, paint on the plastic a little at a time.

Fitting a bald cap

1 Gel the hair back smoothly. If it is long, wrap it around the head, keeping as close as possible to the contour of the head.

2 If the skin is greasy, put a trace of acetone around the hairline.

3 Place the bald cap on the actor's head, stretching the cap down so that it is tight, with no air trapped inside (see page 47). If you want to change the appearing shape of the head, you can add a foam piece underneath the cap.

4 Slit up the plastic with scissors, cutting on the line that runs behind the ear. Trim around the ear, leaving a section in front of the ear.

5 Stick the cap from the centre of the forehead to around the temples, using spirit gum or surgical adhesive. Use a powder puff to press the cap down. Let it settle for a minute, while the spirit gum dries.

6 Put a little spirit gum behind the ears and stick the cap down, pressing firmly with the powder puff. Make sure that the cap fits closely around the ears. Be careful that the edges do not buckle under. Use a wooden modelling tool to push them flat.

7 Once the cap seems securely stuck down, blend the edges into the skin. With a *plastic cap*, blend the edges with a little acetone (a tissue should always be held underneath the cotton bud to prevent acetone from dropping onto the actor's face). Do not allow the acetone to touch the actor's skin, just the edge of the cap. With a *latex cap* the edges may be blended using a latex-based surgical adhesive called Duo. Apply this thinly on the edge and blend it into the skin.

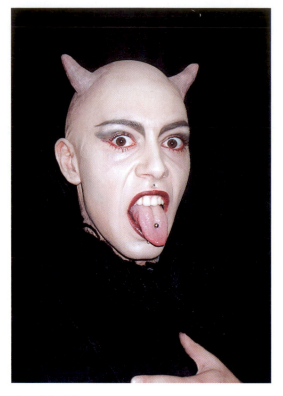

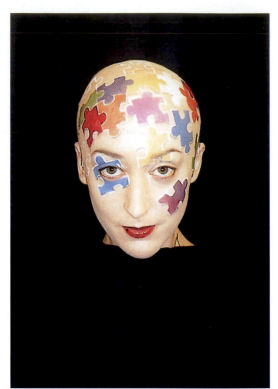

Devil bald cap   Jigsaw bald cap

Tip

Be careful when applying powder. On bald caps the make-up tends to slide.

Applying the make-up to the bald cap

1   Stipple on the colour: red, both dark and light. Use a rubber stipple sponge, or a natural one with plenty of holes in it.

2   Keep the specks of colour this method provides: do not smudge or blend them. Carry the make-up onto the forehead.

3   Powder. Then apply make-up to the rest of the face, according to your design.

Tip

When removing a bald cap, take great care as you loosen the deges. Very often the fine hairs around the hairline can cause pain when they are pulled, especially if the adhesive has glued them to the bald cap.

Colouring the cap

Bald caps are usually given a natural skin tone, to look realistic. For fantasy effects, however, you can use unrealistic colours – green, blue, gold, and so on.

For a realistic look, the bald cap should be stippled with pink and red before the foundation colour, in the same way as you would do with wax noses. Other effects can be achieved by adding hair, for example, clown make-up or a monk's tonsure; or a wig can be applied to create a high forehead, as for a sixteenth-century look (like Elizabeth I).

For fantasy effects, watercolours can be used. For realistic effects, grease or cream is usually stippled on, using a sponge; when using greasepaint, powder must be applied to set it.

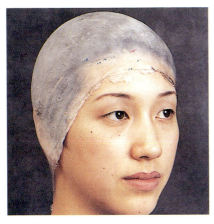

Fitting the bald cap –
The cap has been placed on the
head

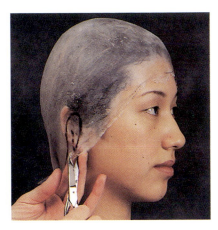

Cutting a section from the
drawn-on ear

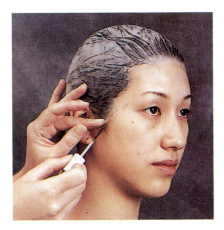

Sticking down the cap

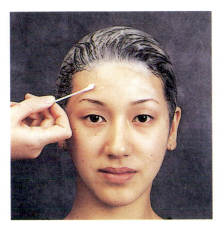

The cap being blended with
acetone

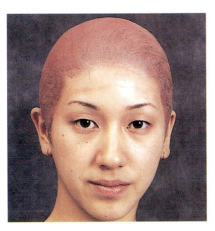

Rose-pink colour has been
stippled onto the cap

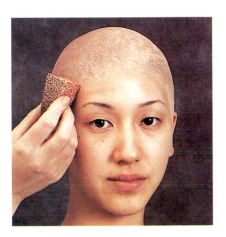

Applying natural camouflage

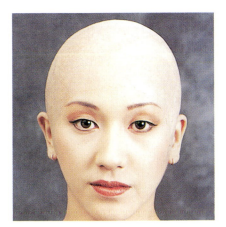

The finished effect

Removing a bald cap

The procedure for removing a bald cap is the same as for removing
all prosthetic pieces, wigs and facial hair. As the *adhesives* vary
according to the materials, however, so do the adhesive *removers*.

Surgical spirit can be used, but use only a little on the tip of a brush.
Work the brush gently under the edge of the bald cap to loosen it.
Always hold a wad of tissues or cottonwool in the other hand, under
the brush. If any of the adhesive remover drips down the forehead,
wipe the skin dry immediately, before the remover reaches the eyes.
This is the most dangerous part of removing the cap.

Once the edges have been loosened, the cap can be easily removed.
When it is off the head you can remove the adhesive from the face
gently and slowly. Then cleanse, tone and moisturise in the usual way.

Acetone should not be used on the face to remove spirit gum. Use it
to clean your brushes and tools.

Adhesive removers

There are many adhesive removers made for use on the skin. *Spirit gum* is sometimes called *mastix*, so some of the removers are called *mastix remover* or *mild mastix remover*. These are in liquid form and gentler than surgical spirit. *Isopropyl alcohol* is used if the adhesive applied was *Dow Corning 355*.

Various adhesive-removing creams are available which are especially kind to the skin and there is an oil called Klene-All which removes most types of adhesive.

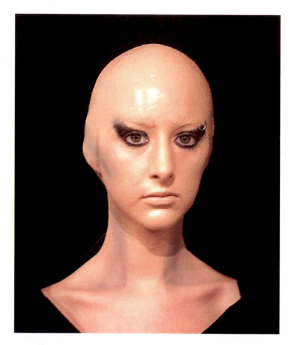

Alien bald cap

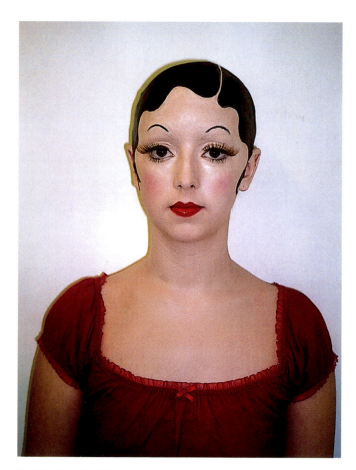

Betty Boo bald cap

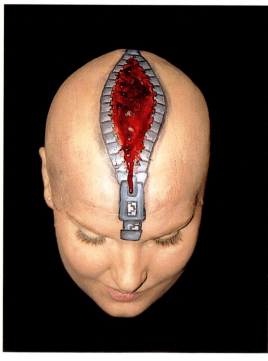

Zip bald cap

Inserting hair into bald caps and prostheses

Hair can be laid onto bald caps and prosthetic pieces, but for tight camera close-ups the hair will look more natural if it is inserted into the latex or plastic.

For this method you need an adapted sewing needle. Remove the tip at the eye end, by rubbing the needle or by cutting it off with pliers. The eye of the needle should present a fork-like appearance. Insert the needle into a knotting hook holder.

The forked needle can now be used to punch individual hairs or tufts of hair into the bald cap or prosthetic appliance. Take the hair in the left hand and hold the needle in the right hand. Catch hold of the hairs with the forked needle and push them through the latex or plastic *from the inside* of the piece. Pull the hair through until you have the desired outside length. The ends can be stuck down with adhesive inside the piece, where they will not show.

This technique works well when hair is needed for prosthetic animal faces, or in an ageing character make-up when you want a few strands of hair across a bald head.

Ageing

Study the faces of older people around you and you will soon see the great variety of ways in which ageing affects people's appearances. Heredity, race, character, lifestyle and environment all play a part. A thin-faced woman who has worked for many years in a city office and suffered recurrent illness may appear pale, gaunt and unhealthy-looking. A well-built, fit old man, on the other hand, who has spent his life out in the sun, rain and wind tending animals on the mountainside, will have a healthy, ruddy complexion, with weathered skin and many wrinkles. The lines on the face will reflect the person's character and temperament. There is a difference between the lines caused by frequent laughter and those caused by illness or bad temper. In *As You Like It* (Act II, scene viii) Shakespeare describes the 'seven ages' of man, from the 'mewling and puking' infant to the 'second childishness' of old age. It's a fine description of the ageing process, which you may like to read.

The creation of a convincing *ageing make-up* will draw on all the skills you have learnt so far. It must be as subtle as straight make-up, but in many respects you are trying to achieve the opposite. Go back to the beginning of your coursework and look again at the anatomy of the face. Recall the drawing of drapery folds and the significance of light and shadow. As we get older our flesh becomes looser and the face starts to drop. In ageing make-up, therefore, you need to put in the shadows that normally you would be trying to conceal, adding bags under the eyes, lines from the nose to the mouth, and so on.

With thin faces it is quite easy to bring out the skull-like effect, by suggesting hollowing at the temples and drooping eyelids. Plumper faces stay looking youthful for longer, but you can add a double chin or sagging flesh, as well as highlights and shading. Hair becomes thicker and coarser in middle age, so you can give a man a dark beardline to take away the smooth look of youth. Broken veins on the face, age spots and greying hair at the temples all help to make the person look older. Don't overdo it: a woman of 45, for example, if she has taken care of her appearance, will not show extensive signs of ageing. Because of the proximity of the audience, ageing make-up for theatre is different to that used in film, as demonstrated throughout this chapter.

Using make-up

Start always from the real face of the person whom you are making up. Study the face; feel the prominences and notice the position and the colour of the natural shadows under the eyes and below the jawline. An overhead light will help you to see where these are. In adding the make-up, your aim is to intensify these shadows.

1   The shading colour must harmonise with the actor's own skin tone. Add a touch of grey to the chosen colour, mixing in a little brown and blue from the basic greasepaint palette. For pale, translucent skins, add a touch of blue or mauve.

2   Only use a foundation if it is necessary to change the skin tone. Apply the shading straight onto the face, emphasising the places where there are shadows already. Look for the age lines, checking that these move with the face. Strengthen the circles under the eyes, the nose-to-mouth lines and the lines at the corners of the mouth. Keep the lines clean – don't let solid make-up smudge into the skin.

3   Add highlighting, blending the edges carefully with a clean brush. On more prominent areas, add more highlighting. Powder lightly between layers. Add the lightest highlights and the darkest shadows last.

4   Try adding a touch of grey and green in the hollows of the face.

5   Tone down the lips with a little blue (to disguise the red of youth). Don't apply much unless your intention is to make the person look ill.

6   If the face is plump and round, emphasise the skin folds: try to make them look as though they have sagged.

7   Whatever the shape of the face, be it plump or thin, you need to 'break up' the jawline and reduce the firmness of youth. On a thinner face, the shadows and highlights will tend to produce a skull-like effect. To produce a double chin on a fuller face, ask the actor to push his or her chin down, then put a shadow in the fold and highlight the bulge where the double chin forms.

8   Try to draw down the shape of the face. Using a stipple sponge, add a stipple of dark red and blue in the highlighted area. With a crimson lake pencil, lightly draw in the broken veins. Blend some of them, with a fine brush.

9 Apply a little red to the upper eyelids, to make the eyes look sore; sparingly outline the bottom eyelids to suggest watery eyes.

10 Paint in liver spots, with brown greasepaint.

11 For an ungroomed look, brush cream or white through the eyebrows and then brush them down.

12 Age the neck by highlighting the bones and placing shading in the hollows and sockets. Blend the highlighting and shading softly at the edges: there must be no hard lines. Keep checking your work by looking in the mirror, turning the face sideways so that you can see the result.

13 Age the hands also: apply highlight to the prominent knuckle bones and along the veins. Shade either side of the veins, and between the fingers.

Equipment and materials

- greasepaints
- powder and brush
- crimson lake pencil
- fine brush

Ageing

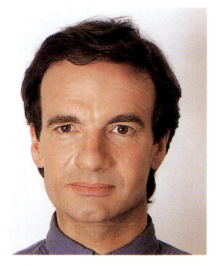 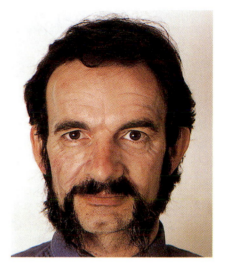

Before   After

Tip

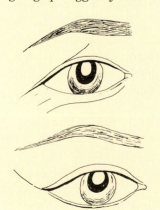

When creating a character which requires ageing, remember that lines going *down* suggest age, and lines going *up* suggest youth.

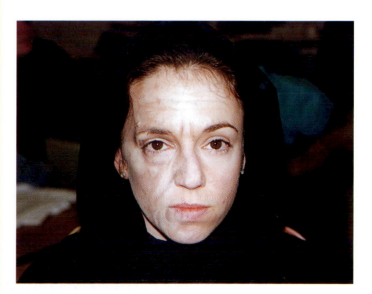

Ageing: for television and film

Activity – Ageing from youth to middle age

Work with a fellow student, ageing him or her from youth to middle age. The guidelines below are for a woman.

1 Apply shadows under the eyes – only in the darkest part of the circles.

2 Tuck your model's chin down, then look in the mirror to find the shadows. Paint shadow in the nose-to-mouth lines – not too much – and then blend the edges.

3 Put a shadow at the corners of the mouth.

4 Ask your model to frown. Put a tiny line where the frown lines appear.

5 Shade in the eye area, concentrating on the inner corners. Add highlight next to the shadows. Use very little make-up or the effect will look too theatrical.

6 Shade softly in the temple depressions. On the forehead, don't paint in lines but highlight the prominences softly and shade the depression.

7 Lightly powder the areas you have made up. (Finish here if you do not wish to create a made-up look.)

8 On top, apply a light liquid foundation. Powder in the usual way.

9 Put on blusher and eyeshadow; strengthen the eyebrows; add eyeliner and mascara.

10 Finish off with carefully applied lipstick – red is a good colour.

Your model should look about 40 years of age.

Equipment and materials

- greasepaints
- powder and brush
- foundation (liquid)
- blusher
- eyeshadow
- eyeliner
- mascara
- lipstick

Variations

To look middle-aged

1 Shade the eyes, from the top of the nose to the eyebrows.
2 Shade under the eyes, gently and lightly.
3 Hollow the cheeks a little more.
4 Add slight nose-to-mouth lines.
5 Break up the cheek muscle by adding a line around the bone.
6 Highlight for puffiness.
7 For a happy character, introduce warm colours into the shading; for a cold character, add cold colours.

To look sixtyish

1 Accentuate the eyebags.
2 Break up the skin tone on the cheeks.
3 Deepen all ageing lines; highlight for puffiness.
4 Hollow the temples and the outside of the eyes.
5 Add a few frown lines and forehead lines.

6 Darken the inner eye sockets.

7 Break up the jawline.

8 Suggest puffiness with highlighting; lighten the cheeks so that they are not a rosy colour.

9 Add lines around the eyes. Whiten these a bit.

10 Add pale ends to the eyebrows, dragging them down.

11 At the centre of the forehead, shade and highlight the prominences.

12 Powder, to set.

13 Stipple in red veins, then stipple on pale colour to break up the skin tone.

14 Stipple on dark brown liver spots.

15 Powder again.

16 Ask the actor to screw up her or his eyes and nose. Tap on light colour with a sponge, to add a few wrinkles.

17 Darken the eyelids, top and bottom. Add more dark lines if necessary.

18 Rework the lines with a clean brush.

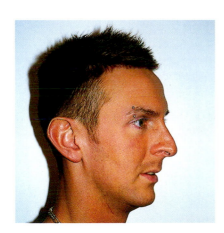

Before

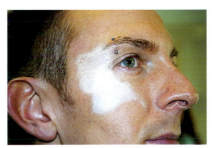

Latex is applied around the eyes

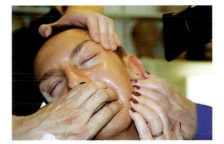

The skin is pulled taut to stretch the latex

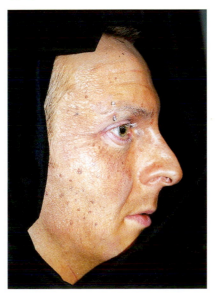

The final result made up with age stipple and age spots using latex (see page 254)

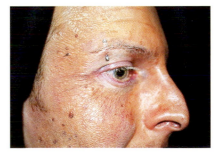

Close-up of latex wrinkles

Ageing for film and television. Make-up by Kulwadee Sangsiri

19 Broken veins can be emphasised with crimson lake-coloured pencil or grease.

20 Add pale eyelids and eye lashes. Darken the sockets of the eyes to close them and bring them down. Use short strokes to create a crepe effect.

21 Make the lips paler.

22 Add a skin-tone coloured base and bleed lipstick into it.

23 Darken under the bottom lip to emphasise the cleft chin.

The highlighting colour 'ivory' is good for ageing.

People often shrink as they get older. One way of creating this effect is for the actor to wear a shirt a size too big.

The face becomes haggard and drawn sometimes, creating the illusion of a bigger nose and extended ear lobes.

Using latex

When painting is inadequate, *latex* is sometimes used to age the face. It does create wrinkles and it gives a very textured effect to the skin. One layer on the eye area can be sufficient to make a middle-aged actor look ten years older without having to age the rest of his face. Care should be taken, however, because latex can easily look mask-like.

Three people are needed when using latex: one to stretch the skin, one to apply the latex and dry the area with a hand-held hairdryer and the third to powder the area before the skin is released. Do not use brushes to put on the latex; they would be ruined.

1 Place a protective wrap around the model's shoulders and tuck a paper tissue around the collar line.

2 Apply barrier cream to the whole eye area. Allow this to sink in.

3 Powder to remove all trace of grease.

4 Pour a little latex into the bowl. If you need to add colour to the latex for use on a dark skin tone, do so now and thoroughly mix it with the latex. You can use dark powder or pigment for this purpose.

5 Working on one area of the face at a time, pull the skin tight with the fingers and, with your small piece of sponge, stipple some of the latex onto the stretched area. Do not overload your sponge piece or the latex will drip into the person's eyes. Discard the sponge pieces after use.

6 Take care to blend the edge of the latex into the skin very thinly. When putting it under the eye to create a pouchy effect, stipple the latex gently beneath the eyes, avoiding the bottom eyelashes; stop at the circle under the eye. Try not to take the latex out beyond the outer corners of the eyes. It would look strange if taken onto the cheekbones.

7 Use the hairdryer, at a good distance from the model's face – put your hand in front of it to test the heat. Take care not to irritate the skin with the dryer set too hot or too cold. Check with the model that he or she is comfortable. (The person stretching the

Equipment and materials

- barrier cream
- liquid latex
- bowl for latex
- powder, powder puff, powder brush
- hairdryer
- sponge cut into small pieces

skin should not relax her hold until after the area has been dried and powdered.) When the latex has become transparent and shiny, it is dry.

8 Powder on top of the dried latex with powder on a powder puff. Brush off the excess powder with a brush. The skin can now be released. It will form into wrinkles. These improve with time as they settle and become part of the model's face.

9 For a more exaggerated set of lines, repeat the procedure – however, one layer is usually enough for close-up work.

10 Clean the bowl by pulling off the dried latex. Remember always to put the tops back on bottles. This is particularly important with latex as the liquid becomes solid very quickly when exposed to the air.

If you apply latex to the whole face, work on small areas, overlapping each one. One layer applied above and one below the eyes is the most commonly used method. You can use the latex all over the face, to get an 'old crone' look.

Wrinkles are formed on the softest parts of the face, where you can stretch the skin easily. The direction in which you stretch the skin will determine the way the wrinkles form. If you pull the skin vertically, the wrinkles will be horizontal; if you stretch horizontally, the lines will be vertical. The neck can be stretched vertically simply by holding the model's head backwards.

If the whole face and neck has been done, the skin on the backs of the hands should be stretched and latex applied. Clench the model's hand into a fist to stretch the skin. (As you will find out, this is a time-consuming task.) To create a good set of wrinkles and so age someone, however, it is usually sufficient to apply latex around the eyes.

Make-up can be applied as usual on the rest of the face. Shading and lighting are not necessary on top of latex. The wrinkles are three-dimensional and create their own shadows.

Ageing with latex

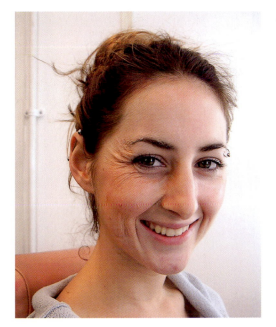

Equipment and materials

- cottonwool
- baby oil or oil-based face cleanser

Removing the latex

1   Use a pad of cottonwool, soaked in warm water and squeezed until damp.

2   Gently lift the edges of the latex with the damp cottonwool. Do not pull the latex off in one piece, especially around the eyes. Instead, gently stretch the skin as you wipe with the cottonwool.

3   Oil can be used also to remove latex. Use baby oil or an oil face cleanser.

Take time and care in removing make-ups like this or you may damage the actor's skin. This type of latex work should be done in quiet, calm conditions. The actor should keep his or her eyes closed when you are working near the eye area.

Ageing for cinematography

In feature films your work will be very evident. On a cinema screen the close-ups are really big: every detail of the actor's face can be seen. The make-up artist's work is much more likely to be noticed and is therefore more open to criticism.

1   When ageing for film, study the person's face and let their natural markings, shadows and highlights be your guide. As before, the best lighting in which to see these shadows is an overhead light which casts straight, natural shadows down the face.

2   First of all, put in your lighting and shading. As well as emphasising the nose-to-mouth lines, the temples and the bridge of the nose, begin to remould the face with patches and shapes of shadow rather than just lines. When you are satisfied, strengthen these so that you have two shades and two highlights.

3   The highlight need not run along the same lines as the shading – it can be thicker or more rounded. Create lines, folds and sunken skin around the side of the face, the jawline and mouth.

4   The eyes don't always need a shaded corner and highlighted brow bone. The emphasis can be on a smaller area, even just a blended line. Remember: a good result often follows from what you don't do. Overworking can easily spoil the effect. Use the mirror constantly and keep studying the natural lines and shape of the face.

5   Once the light and shade is worked in and has graduated folds, the structure is finished. Powder and then texture.

6   Using a sponge, stipple on a red-pink; use your highlight colour to lighten this. Stipple again. You may also use an orange-red. Green can be stippled in around the temples and the beard or stubble line.

7   Age spots can be put on, from the receding hairline to the brow at angles. With red pencil, draw in broken and spider veins. Redden the ears.

8   To age the eyebrows, add grey, coarser hairs (rather than colouring the natural ones).

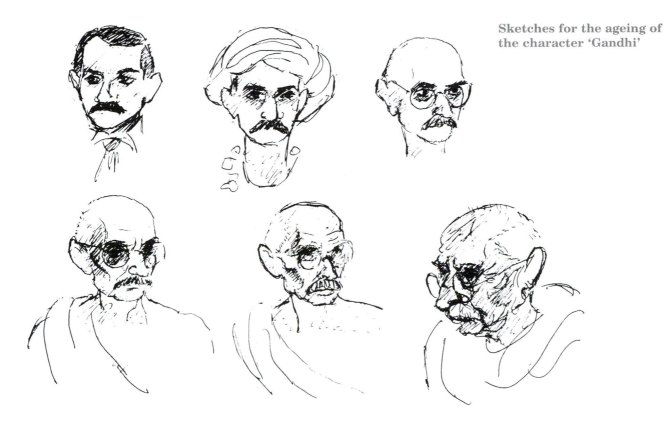

The ageing of the actor, Sir Ben Kingsley, by Tom Smith

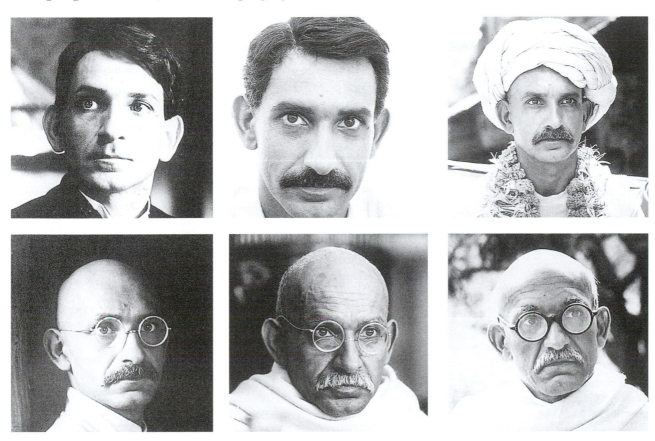

Ageing for theatre. An eigheenth-century ageing make-up for grand opera (note that the audience would be watching from a distance of 6–60 metres)

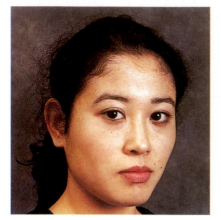

Before

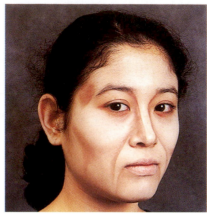

Base and shading lines

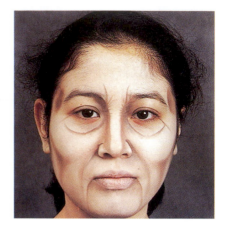

Ageing lines have been added around the eyes

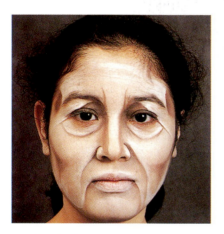

Highlighting and blending

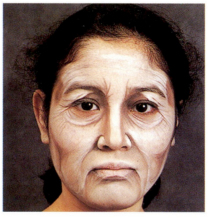

Deepening shadows and strengthening the highlights

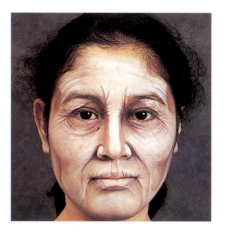

Breaking up the make-up with points of colour, using crimson lake red, blue and white

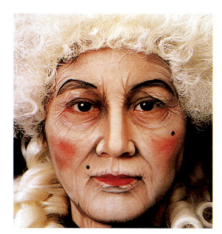

The face is powdered with white talcum and the cheeks heavily rouged. A small mouth is painted in and two beauty spots added with a black pencil

Activity

Using sketches and photographs, compile a reference file. Cut out faces from newspapers and magazines. Place examples of fashion styles with make-up together in one section; in another, collate pictures of elderly faces. Shapes of noses, mouths, eyes, chins and so on are all useful.

As you progress in make-up, add to this file. You will never finish collecting pictures as long as you work. Professional make-up artists refer to their reference files constantly. Start yours today!

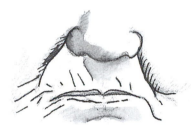

An ageing mouth

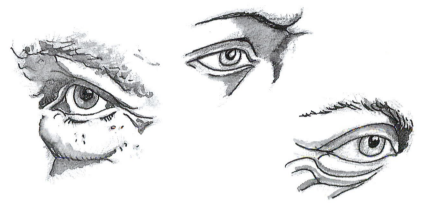

Ageing eyes

Epilogue

When an actor has thought through, developed and rehearsed his or her part, when the director has given assistance and constructive criticism concerning how the role fits within the film or play, when they are in accord, the lighting is arranged and the costumes are ready, then the only remaining contribution to a good or even a great performance is the visual appearance of the performer.

This is in the hands of the make-up artist. If the make-up is true, in combination with the feelings of the actor it will afford the audience a true appreciation of the production.

Glossary

acetone A liquid solvent which melts plastic. It can be used for cleaning hair lace, but should never be used directly on the skin. Commonly it is used for removing nail varnish. It is available from chemists.

adhesive A means of sticking different surfaces together. Various types are available, for use with wig hair laces, eyelashes, prosthetics and so on. Adhesives are available from theatrical suppliers and chemists.

ageing stipple A latex product used for wrinkled ageing effects. It can be obtained in different flesh colours from theatrical make-up suppliers.

alginate A dental impression material used in lifecasting. It is available from dental suppliers.

analysing a character The technique of determining the make-up requirements of an actor, according to the script.

appliances Prosthetic pieces which are applied to the actor's face or body.

aquacolour A cake make-up which is grease-free and is applied with a damp sponge or brush. It is used for body make-up and fantasy painting.

blending The technique of graduating the intensity of the colour from its strongest tone to its lightest until it disappears into the natural skin tone.

block A head-shaped template for use in wig work, or a beard-shaped one for facial hair work. It can be malleable, wooden or plastic and is available from hairdressing suppliers.

blocking pins Pins used to attach wigs to blocks. They are available from hairdressing suppliers.

breaking down The technique of applying make-up to achieve a natural weathered or discoloured effect according to the action and location, such as for a coal mine, desert, fight scene, or the aftermath of an earthquake.

break down the script The technique of going through a script systematically in order to organise crowd scenes, locations, continuity needs and changes of make-up and hairstyles.

camouflage make-up Ointment-based creams used for covering scars and other remedial work, available from chemists and theatrical make-up suppliers.

castor oil An oil used with make-up for colouring prosthetic pieces.

chamois leather A piece of leather used in attaching hair-lace wigs, beards and all facial hair. It is available from paint or hardware stores.

Chinese brushes Long, pointed brushes for watercolour painting to produce various effects, including marbling.

compressed powders Powders in a variety of colours, shiny or matt, used as colouring for the eyelids (eyeshadows) or for the cheeks (blushers or rouge). They are also used for colouring eyebrows. Available from make-up suppliers.

contact lenses Lenses used for special effects in films or television productions, to change the eye colour. They must be supplied and fitted by a qualified optician.

continuity The technique of achieving a seamless sequence in productions (which are usually filmed out of order) by making sure that the make-up and hair 'match' the preceding and following shots.

double knotting The technique of using two knots together when knotting hair onto a foundation net.

drawing mats Mats used in postiche work for drawing hair.

dressing out a wig The technique of styling the hair with tools such as rollers, tongs, a hairdryer and brushes to produce the finished effect.

duplicating material A material used for taking impressions, as in lifecasting. Dentists' alginate is used, which is available from dental suppliers.

eyelashes, false Lashes used for extra emphasis on the eyes, available in different lengths and thicknesses. They are trimmed, then applied with a latex adhesive.

face powder Powder used over the foundation to set it and to reduce shine. An all-purpose translucent loose powder is enough to suit all occasions, though many colours are available. Face powder in compact form (compressed face powder) can be applied directly to the skin without a base, or used on top of the foundation base to give a matt finish.

fantasy make-up A make-up that does not look natural. It might be bizarre or stylised, such as for a witch or a statue.

flash The edge of a prosthetic piece made of gelatine or foam latex. The flash is sculpted prior to casting to provide an overflow for the foam or gelatine.

foundation (face) The make-up base used to achieve a complexion in the desired colour.

foundation (wigs) The base, made out of net, into which hair is knotted to make a wig.

gelatine A material used for directly applied casualty effects and for making prosthetic pieces.

glycerine A material mixed with water and used to simulate perspiration and tears. A spoonful of glycerine mixed with a bottle of rosewater is a good refresher or toner for dry skins. Glycerine is available from chemists.

hackle A tool used in combing and mixing loose hair. Constructed of metal spikes set in a wooden block, it is rather like a miniature bed of nails.

hair, human Hair used for making fine wigs, toupees and other hairpieces.

hair, synthetic Hair generally used for stylised wigs and normally made into weft for wigs, beards and moustaches.

hair, yak Coarse yak hair is used for laying on directly applied hair for beards and moustaches.

hair lace A net-like material, also called ventilating net, into which hair is knotted for many types of postiche.

Head block Block used in making bald caps.

highlighting The technique of using a light colour to make a feature more obvious.

Karo syrup A type of syrup, used in the manufacture of artificial blood. It is available from specialist grocers.

knotting hooks Hooks attached to needles, used for inserting hair into gauze when making postiche.

latex A natural rubber in milky-white foam, available in varying densities. It is used for creating wrinkles in ageing make-up; in casualty effects, for peeling skin and the like; and in making bald caps and filling moulds in prosthetic work.

laying a beard The technique of making a beard by applying loose hair directly onto the face.

laying on hair The technique of sticking loose hair directly onto the face and then dressing it with tongs.

lifecasting The technique of taking an impression of the actor's face or body and casting it in stone.

lifecasting, sectional The technique of taking an impression of a section or piece of the actor's face or body and casting it in stone.

look-alike The character make-up required to make the actor look like someone else.

luminous make-up Fluorescent make-up for fantasy make-up effects, for use under ultraviolet lights. It is available from theatrical make-up suppliers as a cream, a liquid or a gel.

modelling clay Clay used for sculpting features in prosthetic work. It is available from pottery and artists' suppliers.

modelling tools Tools used for building and modelling in clay, plastic and wax. Sculpting tools and dentists' tools are useful to the make-up artist.

modelling with wax The technique of building up a natural feature and changing its shape using wax directly applied to the face or body.

mortician's wax Wax used for modelling directly onto the face, when blocking out eyebrows, changing the shape of the nose, and so on.

moustaches wax A coloured wax used to curl the ends of moustaches.

pancake A cake make-up which is grease-free. It was first made by Max Factor.

panstik A cream stick make-up base, also available in paintbox-style containers, obtained from the theatrical make-up shops.

pencils Wooden pencils with soft grease lead, used for colouring eyebrows and outlining eyes and lips.

plaster A material used for making positive and negative moulds in prosthetic work. It is available from dental or artists' suppliers.

plaster bandage Bandage used to reinforce the impression when lifecasting.

plastic A material used in liquid form to paint layers when making bald caps and prosthetic pieces. Glatzan is a well-known make available from theatrical make-up shops. Plastic should never be used directly on the face.

plastic scar material A material in tube form used for modelling scars and the like directly onto the skin. Although especially formulated for use on the skin, this material should always be tested on the back of the actor's hand first, in case of irritation.

plastic spray An artificial latex spray used for setting facial hair when making hair on a block. It is not for facial use.

plastilene A material used for modelling in prosthetic work. Although not as good as clay, unlike clay it does not need wetting. It is available from artists' suppliers.

powder brush A soft brush used for removing excess powder from the face.

rubber-mask greasepaint A castor-oil-based product, available in various colours, used for painting on top of latex.

sealer A material used on top of wax, nose putty and prosthetic pieces before applying make-up.

shading The technique of using a darker colour to make a feature less obvious.

spirit gum The adhesive most commonly used in attaching wigs, beards, moustaches, bald caps and the like. It is available from theatrical make-up shops.

standing by Staying near the actors on the set, ready to retouch the make-up when necessary.

stippling The technique of using an open-pored sponge and applying make-up with a dabbing movement in order to provide a textured effect.

straight make-up The technique of defining and correcting a face with make-up.

stubble paste Wax in stick form, used on the face before applying chopped-up hair to create a beard stubble.

test shots (cinematography) The filming and viewing on a screen of the lighting, hair, make-up and costumes, to try them out.

test shots (photography) Photographs taken by the photographer, model and make-up artist working together unpaid to produce pictures for their portfolios.

tong heater An electronic heater for heating iron tongs used in dressing postiche.

tongs Iron tools heated up to dress hair.

toning down a colour The technique of making the colour less bright by adding a complementary one, such as toning down red by adding green.

toning down a period look The technique of making a look more modern.

tooth enamel A material used for painting the teeth. It is available in white, cream, nicotine, yellow, black, gold and silver from theatrical make-up shops.

watercolour brushes Brushes used for applying sealer, collodion, spirit gum, acrylic paints, latex and cap plastic. They should be cleaned in the appropriate solvent immediately after use.

waterproofing the make-up The technique of protecting the make-up for filming in water.

waxing out The technique of using a layer of wax to cover a feature such as the eyebrows before applying make-up.

wig stand A stand used to hold a wig or moustache block while dressing postiche. Stands are available either free standing or as a shorter version that clamps to a workbench or table.

witch hazel A material used for blending the edges of gelatine pieces. A spoonful mixed in a bottle of rosewater makes a good refresher or toner for greasy skin. Witch hazel is available from chemists.

Recommended reading

Allsworth, Joyce (1985) *Skin Camouflage*. Stanley Thornes.

Baker, Patricia (1993) *Wigs and Make-up for Theatre, Television and Film*. Butterworth Heinemann.

Baker, Patricia (1991) *Fashions of a Decade: the 1950s*. Batsford.

Baygan, Lee (1984) *Make-up for Theatre and Television*. A & C Black.

Baygan, Lee (1988) *Techniques of Three-Dimensional Make-up*. Watson-Guptill.

Buchman, Herman (1973) *Film and Television Make-up*. Watson-Guptill.

Buchman, Herman (1989) *Stage Make-up*. Watson-Guptill.

Cameron, Patrick and Wadeson, Jacki (2001) *Dressing Long Hair*. Thomson Learning.

Corson, Richard (1972) *Fashions in Make-up*. Peter Owen.

Corson, Richard (1986) *Stage Make-up*. Peter Owen.

Corson, Richard (1991) *Fashions in Hair*. Peter Owen.

Gray, Henry F.R.S. (2001) *Gray's Anatomy*. Serpents Tail.

Green, Martin *et al.* (1994) *Professional Hairdressing*. Macmillan.

Henderson, Stephanie (1991) *Basic Hairdressing level 2*. Thornes.

Hogarth, Burne (1989) *Drawing the Human Head*. Watson-Guptill.

Innes, Jocasta (1981) *Paint Magic*. Frances Lincoln Publishers.

Kehoe, Vincent J.R. (1985) *The Technique of the Professional Make-up Artist for Film, Television and Stage*. Focal Press.

Kehoe, Vincent J.R. (1991) *Special Make-up Effects*. Butterworth Heinemann.

McDowell, Colin (1998) *Galliano*. Orion.

Mulvey, Kate and Richards, Melissa (2000) *Decades of Beauty 1890s–1990s: The Changing Image of Women*. Hamlyn.

Nunn, Joan (1990) *Fashion in Costume 1200–1980*. Herbert Press.

Palladino, Leo (1989) *The Principles and Practice of Hairdressing*. Macmillan.

Palladino, Leo (1991) *Hairdressing – The Foundations*. Macmillan.

Palladino, Leo and Hunt, June (1992) *The Nail File*. Macmillan.

Saper, Chris (2001) *Painting Beautiful Skin Tones with Colour & Light*. David & Charles.

Savini, Tom (1987) *Grande Illusions*. Imagine Inc.

Sennett, Tom (1983) *Great Hollywood Movies*. Abradale Press.

Smith, Dick (1986) *Dick Smith's Do-It-Yourself Monster Make-up Hand book*. Random House.

Wickham, Glynne (1985) *A History of the Theatre*. Phaidon.

Index

PITTSBURGH FILMMAKERS
477 MELWOOD AVENUE
PITTSBURGH, PA 15213